THOMSON DELMAR LEARNING'S
CASE STUDY SERIES

Pharmacology

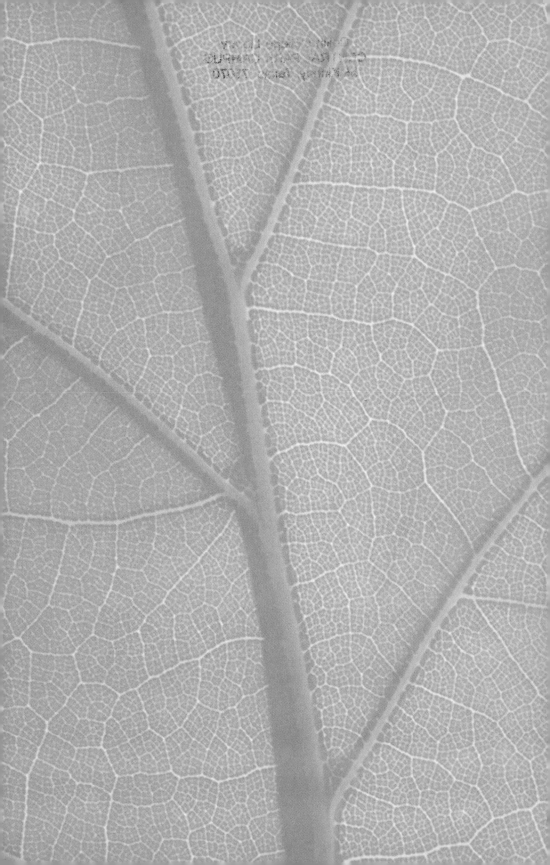

THOMSON DELMAR LEARNING'S
CASE STUDY SERIES

Pharmacology

Hyacinth C. Martin

THOMSON
—*—
DELMAR LEARNING

Australia   Canada   Mexico   Singapore   Spain   United Kingdom   United States

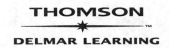

THOMSON

DELMAR LEARNING

Thomson Delmar Learning's Case Study Series: Pharmacology
by Hyacinth C. Martin, BSN, MA, MSEd, MPS, RNBC

**Vice President,
Health Care Business Unit:**
William Brottmiller

Director of Learning Solutions:
Matthew Kane

Acquisitions Editor:
Maureen Rosener

Product Manager:
Elizabeth Howe

Editorial Assistant:
Chelsey Iaquinta

Marketing Director:
Jennifer McAvey

Marketing Manager:
Michele McTighe

Marketing Coordinator:
Danielle Pacella

Production Director:
Carolyn Miller

Content Project Manager:
Jessica McNavich

Library of Congress Cataloging-in-Publication Data

Martin, Hyacinth C.
    Pharmacology/Hyacinth C. Martin.
        p. ; cm. —
    (Thomson Delmar Learning's case study series)
    Includes bibliographical references.
    ISBN 1-4018-3523-6 (pbk. : alk. paper)
    1. Clinical pharmacology—Case studies. 2. Nursing—Case studies.
    I. Title. II. Series. [DNLM:
    1. Pharmacology, Clinical—methods— Case Reports. 2. Pharmacology, Clinical—methods—Nurses' Instruction. 3. Drug Therapy— nursing—Case Reports. 4. Drug Therapy—nursing—Nurses' Instruction.

QV 38 M3814p 2007]
RM301.28.M393 2007
610.73—dc22   2006007601

Notice to the Reader

Publisher does not warrant or guarantee any of the products described herein or perform any independent analysis in connection with any of the product information contained herein. Publisher does not assume, and expressly disclaims, any obligation to obtain and include information other than that provided to it by the manufacturer.

The reader is expressly warned to consider and adopt all safety precautions that might be indicated by the activities described herein and to avoid all potential hazards. By following the instructions contained herein, the reader willingly assumes all risks in connection with such instructions.

The publisher makes no representations or warranties of any kind, including but not limited to, the warranties of fitness for particular purpose or merchantability, nor are any such representations implied with respect to the material set forth herein, and the publisher takes no responsibility with respect to such material. The publisher shall not be liable for any special, consequential, or exemplary damages resulting, in whole or part, from the readers' use of, or reliance upon, this material.

Contents

Reviewers

Mary Beth Kiefner, RN, MS
Nursing Program Director
Nursing Faculty, Illinois Central College
East Peoria, Illinois

Joan Piper Mader, RN, MSN
Associate Professor or Nursing
College of the Mainland
Texas City, Texas

Darla R. Ura, MA, RN, APRN, BC
Clinical Associate Professor
Department of Adult and Elder Health Nursing
School of Nursing, Emory University
Atlanta, Georgia

Mari A. Smith, DSN, RN, CCRN
Professor
School of Nursing, Middle Tennessee State University
Murfreesboro, Tennessee

Preface

Thomson Delmar Learning's Case Study Series was created to encourage nurses to bridge the gap between content knowledge and clinical application. The products within the series represent the most innovative and comprehensive approach to nursing case studies ever developed. Each title has been authored by experienced nurse educators and clinicians who understand the complexity of nursing practice as well as the challenges of teaching and learning. All of the cases are based on real-life clinical scenarios and demand thought and "action" from the nurse. Each case brings the user into the clinical setting, and invites her to utilize the nursing process while considering all of the variables that influence the client's condition and the care to be provided. Each case also represents a unique set of variables, to offer a breadth of learning experiences and to capture the reality of nursing practice. To gauge the progression of a user's knowledge and critical thinking ability, the cases have been categorized by difficulty level. Every section begins with basic cases and proceeds to more advanced scenarios, thereby presenting opportunities for learning and practice for both students and professionals.

All of the cases have been expert reviewed to ensure that as many variables as possible are represented in a truly realistic manner and that each case reflects consistency with realities of modern nursing practice.

How to Use This Book

Every case begins with a table of variables that are encountered in practice, and that must be understood by the nurse in order to provide appropriate care to the client. Categories of variables include age, gender, setting, culture, ethnicity, cultural considerations, preexisting conditions, coexisting conditions, communication considerations, disability considerations, socioeconomic considerations, spiritual considerations, pharmacological considerations, psychosocial considerations, legal considerations, ethical considerations, alternative therapy, prioritization considerations, and delegation considerations. If a case involves a variable that is considered to have a significant impact on care, the specific variable is included in the table. This allows the user an "at a glance" view of the issues that will need to be considered to provide care to the client in the scenario. The table of variables is followed by a presentation of the case, including the history of the client, current condition, clinical setting, and professionals involved. A series of questions follows each case that ask the user to consider how she would handle the issues presented within the scenario.

Organization

Cases are grouped according to body system. Within each part, cases are organized by difficulty level from easy, to moderate, to difficult. These classifications are somewhat subjective, but they are based upon a developed standard. In general, difficulty level has been determined by the number of variables that impact the case and the complexity of the client's condition. Colored tabs are used to allow the user to distinguish the difficulty levels more easily. A comprehensive table of variables is also provided for reference, to allow the user to quickly select cases containing a particular variable of care.

While every effort has been made to group cases into the most applicable body system, the scope of many of the cases may include more than one body system. In such instances, the case will still only appear in the section for one of the body systems addressed. The cases are fictitious; however, they are based on actual problems and/or situations the nurse will encounter. Any resemblance to actual cases or individuals is coincidental.

Praise for Thomson Delmar Learning's Case Study Series

"[This text's] strength is the large variety of case studies – it seemed to be all inclusive. Another strength is the extensiveness built into each case study. You can almost see this person as they enter the ED because of the descriptions that are given."

—MARY BETH KIEFNER, RN, MS
Nursing Program Director/Nursing Faculty,
Illinois Central College

"The cases . . . reflect the complexity of nursing practice. They are an excellent way to refine critical thinking skills."

—DARLA R. URA, MA, RN, APRN, BC
Clinical Associate Professor, Department of Adult
and Elder Health Nursing, School of Nursing,
Emory University

"This text does an excellent job of reflecting the complexity of nursing practice."

—VICKI NEES, RNC, MSN, APRN-BC
Associate Professor, Ivy Tech State College

". . . the case studies are very comprehensive and allow the undergraduate student an opportunity to apply knowledge gained in the classroom to a potentially real clinical situation."

—TAMELLA LIVENGOOD, APRN, BC, MSN, FNP
Nursing Faculty, Northwestern Michigan College

"These cases and how you have approached them definitely stimulate the students to use critical-thinking skills. I thought the questions asked really pushed the students to think deeply and thoroughly."

—JOANNE SOLCHANY, PhD, ARNP, RN, CS
Assistant Professor, Family & Child Nursing,
University of Washington, Seattle

"The use of case studies is pedagogically sound and very appealing to students and instructors. I think that some instructors avoid them because of the challenge of case development. You have provided the material for them."

—NANCY L. OLDENBURG, RN, MS, CPNP
Clinical Instructor, Northern Illinois University

"[The author] has done an excellent job of assisting students to engage in critical thinking. I am very impressed with the cases, questions and content. I rarely ask that students buy more than one . . . book . . . but, in this instance, I can't wait until this book is published."

—DEBORAH J. PERSELL, MSN, RN, CPNP
Assistant Professor, Arkansas State University

"This is a groundbreaking book. . . . This book should be a required text for all undergraduate and graduate nursing programs and should be well-received by faculty."

—JANE H. BARNSTEINER, PHD, RN, FAAN
Professor of Pediatric Nursing, University of
Pennsylvania School of Nursing

About the Author

Hyacinth C. Martin was first influenced by her elementary school teacher in choosing nursing as a career. However, the major influential persons in her choice of nursing as a career were nurses who wore white uniforms, white shoes, including nursing hats, and who seemed to have generated the highest respect from those they came in contact with. Hyacinth's nursing career includes staff nurse experiences on medical-surgical units, head nurse/nurse manager for medical-surgical units and critical-care units, administrative nursing supervisor, community nursing, and administrative nursing supervisor in long-term care agencies. Her academic experiences include teaching theory and clinical in a Licensed Practical Nursing program, a Baccalaureate Degree Program and at present in an Associate Degree program. In 1999, Hyacinth was a guest speaker on WMBC-TV (Channel 63, Newton, NJ), discussing issues pertaining to multiculturalism, with focus on multi-cultural marriage and its effects on the family.

Publications include two articles for a nursing journal, one manuscript for Continuing Medical Education Resource, and part of a chapter on the endocrine system, published by Thomson Delmar Learning. She has also reviewed a chapter in *Pharmacology for Nursing Care*, Richard A. Lehne (5th ed.), and revised *PowerPoint for Pharmacology for Nursing Care* (6th ed.) and an instructor's manual. She was a contributor for *Gerontological Nursing Textbook* (2006), P. A. Tabloski.

Her contributions to education include recent presentations: "Pulmonary Tuberculosis: Controlling the Transmission of the Disease," at PACE University Conference; "Civic Society, Environmental Responsibility, & Sustainable Development in the United States & Brazil," presented at the Manhattan Veteran's Hospital Medical Center Conference, New York; and "The Effective Use of Unfractionated and Fractionated Heparin Therapy to Patients at Risk for Thrombus Formation" and "Nurse's Nurturing Nurses," presented at Lincoln Hospital Medical Center, New York.

Achievements

Hyacinth Martin was recognized in Who's Who Among American Teachers for four successive years. A current recipient of a PSC-CUNY grant for research on Gender and Career Choice in Nursing, she is a full-time tenured professor in the nursing program at Borough of Manhattan Community College/The City University of New York. Her passion in teaching is to assist in the success of students who enroll in the nursing program at Borough of Manhattan Community College.

Hyacinth's other contributions (along with her husband's) to the welfare of others include adopting a basic school in one of the West Indian islands, and sponsoring a nursing student in Davao City, Philippines. Hyacinth earned a BSN degree and a Master's Degree in Career Guidance and Counseling from Lehman College, a Master's Degree in Nursing Administration from Columbia University, and a Master's Degree in Urban Education/Theology from NYACK College, New York. She is currently pursuing a doctoral degree in theology.

Acknowledgments

I want to express my sincere thanks to Elizabeth Howe, Product Manager, for the professional manner in which she communicated with me both verbally and by e-mail. I also want to thank the entire editorial staff at Thomson Delmar Learning for guidance in writing this text. I wish to record my thanks to the accuracy reviewer, Bonita E. Broyles, RN, BSN, EdD. Your excellent guidance removed much of the stress that writing the text generated. A special thanks to Reverend Florentina Lapsey and Professor Louise Green for their constant prayers as I pursued the task of research and writing the text. I am grateful to Dr. David Ephraim for his encouragement, and the many hours spent making sure computers and laptops were functioning, and lost content restored. Lastly, thank you, Professor Boyle-Egland for that special moment of support as the text was entering its final stage.

This book is dedicated to:

My granddaughter, Nardia – May you also become the author of many books.

My husband, Frederick, a retired registered nurse himself, in recognition of all that I owe him for his patience and understanding as he took on the responsibility of most of the household chores, to enable me to accomplish this goal. It is my hope and prayer that this modest work will assist nursing students to better understand the content of medical-surgical nursing and, in so doing, help them to appreciate more of the incredible writings of nurse authors.

Hyacinth C. Martin

Comprehensive Table
of Variables

CASE STUDY	GENDER	AGE	SETTING	ETHNICITY/CULTURE	LIFESTYLE	PREEXISTING CONDITIONS	COEXISTING CONDITIONS	LIFESTYLE	COMMUNICATION	DISABILITY	SOCIOECONOMIC	SPIRITUAL/RELIGION	PHARMACOLOGIC	PSYCHOSOCIAL	LEGAL	ETHICAL	ALTERNATIVE THERAPY	PRIORITIZATION	DELEGATION
Part One: The Digestive and Urinary Systems																			
1	F	40	Outpatient clinic	Black American	Works 5 days per week in a day care center as a teacher's assistant	x	x	x			x	x	x	x			x	x	x
2	M	56	Clinic	White American	Consumes only 1 meal per day for several years; Consumes 3 cans of beer daily	x	x	x			x	x	x	x		x		x	x
3	F	45	Hospital	Native American	Restaurant cashier	x	x	x		x	x	x	x	x		x	x	x	x
4	M	60	Hospital	White American	Unemployed; Previously employed by fire department	x	x	x			x	x	x	x				x	x
Part Two: The Respiratory and Immune Systems																			
1	M	65	Adult home/hospital	White American	Retired bus operator for private company	x	x	x		x	x	x	x	x		x	x	x	x
2	F	30	Hospital asthma clinic	Hispanic	Full-time college student	x		x	x		x	x	x	x				x	
3	F	70	Nursing home to hospital	Black American	Retired housewife	x		x			x	x	x	x				x	x
4	F	40	Hospital	Black American/West Indian descent	Registered nurse/nurse educator	x	x	x		x	x	x	x	x	x	x	x	x	x
Part Three: The Cardiovascular and Lymphatic Systems																			
1	M	32	Office	Asian/Phillipines	College student	x	x	x	x	x	x	x	x	x	x	x	x	x	x

#	Sex	Age	Location	Ethnicity	Description
2	F	45	Office	White American	Works as an executive secretary in a law firm / Plays the piano for Sunday school / Drinks at least 6 cups of coffee daily for several years
3	M	48	Home	Black American	Bank manager, works 5 days per week
4	M	60	ER	White American	Electrical engineer
5	M	72	Hospital	Black American	Owner of several rental homes
6	F	65	Hospital	Black American	Self-employed hair designer

Part Four: The Nervous System

#	Sex	Age	Location	Ethnicity	Description
1	F	43	Office	Black American	Director, Licensed Practical Nurse program
2	F	52	Hospital	Black American	Employed full time as a registered nurse in a community clinic / Uses hair dyes to color hair occasionally
3	M	70	Office	White American	Retired postal employee

Part Five: The Endocrine System

#	Sex	Age	Location	Ethnicity	Description
1	F	50	Office	Black American	Elementary school teacher
2	F	40	Hospital	American/Asian	Intake clerk
3	F	68	Hospital	Hispanic American	Retired principal, elementary school

Part Six: Other Body Systems: Musculoskeletal and Reproductive

#	Sex	Age	Location	Ethnicity	Description
1	M	58	Urology clinic	Black American	Licensed plumber
2	F	42	Outpatient	White American	Housewife
3	F	52	Home	Black American/West Indian	Ordained minister / Early retirement as laboratory technician

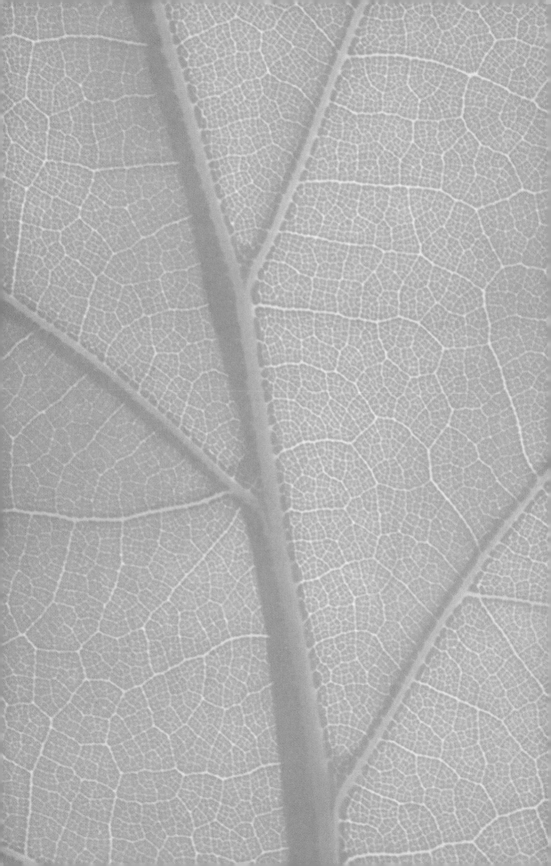

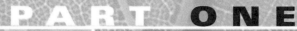

PART ONE

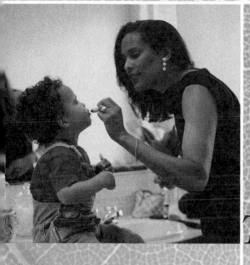

The Digestive and Urinary Systems

CASE STUDY 1

Iron Deficiency Anemia

GENDER

  F

AGE

  40

SETTING

- Outpatient clinic of a medical center

ETHNICITY/CULTURE

- Black American

PREEXISTING CONDITIONS

- Gastric ulcers
- Inflammatory bowel disease

COEXISTING CONDITIONS

- History of excessive menstrual bleeding
- Celiac disease
- Gastrectomy

LIFESTYLE

- Works five days per week in a day care center as a teacher's assistant

COMMUNICATION

DISABILITY

SOCIOECONOMIC

- Low

SPIRITUAL/RELIGIOUS

- Baptist
- Strong faith in prayer

PHARMACOLOGIC

- Acetaminophen (Tylenol)
- Enteric-coated ferrous sulfate (Feosol)

PSYCHOSOCIAL

- Anxiety

LEGAL

ETHICAL

ALTERNATIVE THERAPY

- SSS Tonic, a high-potency iron/B supplement
- Women's natural herbal tonic

PRIORITIZATION

- Nutritional assessment
- Send specimen for serum lab

DELEGATION

- RN
- Client education

EASY

THE DIGESTIVE AND URINARY SYSTEMS

Level of difficulty: Easy

Overview: This case involves a thorough assessment of the client's economic constraints that could prevent dietary meals that include food sources that are high in iron. It also involves reviewing a 24-hour nutritional intake of the client and history of anorexia or lack of interest in food preparation.

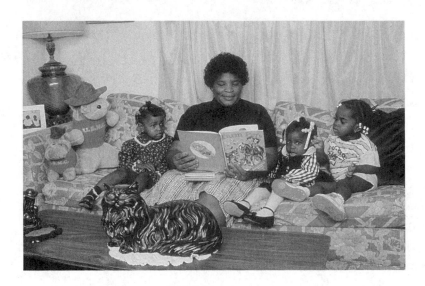

Client Profile

Ms. S is a 40-year-old single parent with children ages 10 and 5 years old. She is a teacher's assistant at a day care center. Ms. S reports that her working days begin at 5:30 a.m., Monday through Friday. Her 5-year-old child attends the day care center where she is employed; the 10-year-old attends a public school in their community. Ms. S is seen by a nurse practitioner (NP) at a community health center clinic because of her concerns of glossitis, cheilitis, and unusual dryness at the corners of her mouth. The NP collects data and completes the history, physical nutritional screening, and assessment. Ms. S also complains of unexplained fatigue, even after seven hours of sleep. She is concerned about the unexplained fatigue because she has been taking a "high potency tonic drink and a natural herbal tonic supplement for women" for several months. Her vital signs are:

Blood pressure: 130/78
Pulse: 78 and regular
Respirations: 18
Temperature: 98.6° F

Case Study

Ms. S is later seen by a health care provider in the health clinic and undergoes further interview and assessment. She is sent to the community hospital outpatient clinic for the following serum labs: hematocrit (Hct), hemoglobin

(Hgb), iron transferrin, total binding iron capacity, and peripheral blood smear. The results of the serum labs are:

Hematocrit (Hct): 28%
Hemoglobin (Hgb): 12 g/dL
Serum iron: 85 ug/dL
Transferrin: 220 mg/dL
Total iron binding capacity: 300 ug/dL

The peripheral blood smear reveals some abnormal types of red blood cells (RBCs), and stool for occult blood is negative. A health care provider at the hospital's outpatient clinic reviewed the labs with Ms. S and suggested a bone marrow examination, which the health care provider explains would confirm a diagnosis. Ms. S signs a written consent, witnessed by a nurse, and the bone marrow aspiration is done. The client is allowed to rest for one hour while the specimen is examined. The findings reveal small RBCs and a decrease in RBCs and Hct, which, when combined with the laboratory results, confirmed the diagnosis of iron deficiency anemia (IDA). Ms. S is discharged to home.

Questions

1. Explain the pathophysiology of IDA.

2. Discuss the prevalence of IDA.

3. Discuss classic manifestations of IDA.

4. Discuss specific diagnostic findings in IDA.

5. Discuss bone marrow aspiration and the nurse's role for this procedure.

6. Discuss radiographic studies that may be done for persons 50 years and older who have IDA.

7. What are the purposes for the prescribed orders?

8. What are the most common adverse reactions, drug-to-drug interactions, drug-to-food/herbal interactions for the prescribed medications?

9. Discuss client education for IDA.

10. Explain nursing implications for clients with IDA.

Questions and Suggested Answers

1. **Explain the pathophysiology of IDA.** IDA, also classified as one of the hypoproliferative anemias, typically results when the intake of dietary iron is inadequate for hemoglobin synthesis resulting in defective release of iron into the plasma from iron stores, as occurs in chronic inflammation and other chronic disorders. Because the body can store about one-fourth to one-third of its iron, it is not until those stores are depleted that IDA actually begins to develop. Persons with IDA may for a prolonged period of

time have been deficient in the required daily allowance of foods high in iron, resulting in a decreased supply of iron to the developing RBCs, which is a crucial component of the hemoglobin. Because iron is essential to the oxygen-carrying function of hemoglobin, the person often manifests or reports signs of fatigue. Fatigue may be related to the decreased level of hematocrit and hemoglobin, which are measurements of the size and number of RBCs. A decrease in these values is an indication of anemia or blood loss. A decrease in the serum iron is usually due to either decreased nutritional intake or a decrease in iron transferrin, which is a measure of iron status. Iron transferrin is also a trace protein needed for iron absorption and transport. Its decrease may be a primary factor for fatigue in persons with IDA. There may be a decrease in the total iron binding capacity (TIBC), indicating a decrease in iron level since TIBC measures the amount of transferrin available to bind more iron.

2. **Discuss the prevalence of IDA.** IDA is the most common type of anemia in all age groups, and it is the most common type of anemia in the world. More than 500 million people are affected, more commonly in underdeveloped countries where inadequate iron stores can result from inadequate intake of iron (seen with vegetarian diets) and blood loss (e.g., from intestinal hookworm). Iron deficiency is also common in the United States, with common causes of IDA in men and postmenopausal women being bleeding from ulcers, gastritis, inflammatory bowel disease, or gastrointestinal tumors, which interfere with the absorption, thus preventing iron from entering the blood stream in the required amount even though the dietary intake of iron is adequate. In the adult male, IDA is ascribed to blood loss resulting from disease or treatment for disease. The most common cause of IDA in premenopausal women in menorrhagia (excessive menstrual bleeding) and pregnancy with inadequate iron supplementation.

3. **Discuss classic manifestations of IDA.** Classic manifestations include a smooth, sore tongue and angular cheilosis (an ulceration of the corner of the mouth), which may be an indication of glossitis and/or stomatitis. The onset of disease interferes with nail structure resulting in abnormal findings such as soft or brittle nails; ridged nails; normal nails curved, hard, and slightly pink (because of the underlying vascular system) to light brown. In achlorhydria and hypochromic anemia, nails become excessively spoon-shaped and are depressed in the center.

4. **Discuss specific diagnostic findings in IDA.** The most definitive method of establishing the IDA is performing a ***bone marrow aspiration*** examination. Nursing care before the procedure includes reinforcing what the health care provider has told the client, explaining that an informed consent is required; the area to be used will be cleansed with antibacterial solution, and local anesthetic agent will be administered by the health care

provider at the site of insertion. Temporary pain will be felt as the skin is injected with the anesthetic and when the specimen is being drawn out. Positioning of the client is dependent on the site to be used. When the needle is removed, the aspirate is immediately smeared on slides and, when dry, sprayed with a fixative. Immediately upon removal of the needle, the nurse who is assisting the health care provider applies direct pressure to the site. The aspirate is sent to the lab where it is stained to analyze for the presence of iron, which is usually at a low level. There is also a strong correlation between laboratory values measuring iron stores and levels of hemoglobin. The hematocrit (Hct) and hemoglobin (Hgb) are reduced; the mean corpuscular volume (MCV), which measures the size of the RBC, also decreases. Ferritin, which usually reflects iron stores, reveals low serum ferritin levels, but the TIBC is elevated.

5. Discuss bone marrow aspiration and the nurse's role for this procedure. Bone marrow examination (aspiration, biopsy) requires removal of a small sample of the bone marrow by aspiration, needle biopsy, or open surgical biopsy. It is an important part of the evaluation of clients with hematologic diseases. By examination of a bone marrow specimen, the hematologist can fully evaluate hematopoiesis. The nurse's role for bone marrow aspiration includes reinforcing what the health care provider or NP has told the client, checking for a written consent for the procedure, monitoring coagulation studies and reporting abnormal values to the health care provider or NP, informing the health care provider or NP about the client's level of anxiety if present, and obtaining an order for sedative as appropriate. Stress to the client the importance of remaining very still during the procedure and explain the reason for doing so. After the procedure the nurse must monitor blood pressure and pulse, and observe the puncture site for bleeding, reporting as appropriate. The nurse may use ice packs to help control bleeding if not contraindicated. Instruct the client when discharged to home after the aspiration to observe the puncture site for unusual tenderness and erythema, which may indicate infection, and the importance of reporting the findings to the primary care provider. If a mild analgesic such as aspirin or Tylenol is prescribed, teach the client the common side effects and adverse effects of these drugs.

6. Discuss radiographic studies that may be done for persons 50 years and older who have IDA. A *gastroscopy* is done to view the interior of the stomach, to determine if ulcers are present that could be the cause of the low Hct and Hgb. If bleeding is evident, photocoagulation (the use of light energy in the form of ordinary light rays or a laser beam) could be used to control the bleeding. A biopsy of tissue can also be done during the gastroscopy to further aid in diagnosis and treatment. *Colonoscopy* may also be done to provide direct visualization of the entire colon and terminal ileum.

A flexible fiber optic endoscope is inserted as far as the cecum to enhance the view and aid with findings.

The following are prescribed:

- Acetaminophen (Tylenol) 650 mg PO q6h PRN at post-insertion site
- Enteric-coated ferrous sulfate (Feosol) 325 mg PO three times per day
- Return to the outpatient department in two weeks for gastroscopy

7. What are the purposes for the prescribed orders? *Acetaminophen* temporarily relieves mild to moderate pain. It will relieve the mild discomfort that Ms. S may feel for several days at the post-insertion site. It produces analgesia by its action on the peripheral nervous system. *Enteric-coated ferrous sulfate* increases the iron stores in the body because it contains 50–100 mg of elemental iron. Being enteric-coated helps to prevent gastric irritation. Ferrous sulfate also helps to correct erythropoietic abnormalities that may be induced by iron deficiency, and mostly involve the gastrointestinal (GI) tract.

8. What are the most common adverse reactions, drug-to-drug interactions, drug-to-food/herbal interactions for the prescribed medications? The most common adverse reaction of *acetaminophen* is hepatotoxicity. Drug-to-drug interactions may occur with the simultaneous use of high doses of acetaminophen, and alcohol may increase the risk of bleeding with warfarin. Simultaneous use with sulfinpyrazone, isoniazid, rifampin, rifabutin, phenytoin, barbiturates, and carbamazepine may increase the risk of acetaminophen-induced liver damage. The simultaneous use with propranolol decreases *acetaminophen* metabolism and may increase toxic effects. Simultaneous use with lamotrigine, zidovudine, and loop diuretics may decrease their effects.

The most common adverse effects of *enteric-coated ferrous sulfate* are dose dependent. They are nausea, pyrosis (heartburn), bloating, constipation, and diarrhea. Drug-to-drug interactions may occur with the simultaneous use of antacids, which may reduce the absorption of iron. The simultaneous use of levofloxacin reduces iron absorption. The simultaneous use of tetracycline decreases the absorption of ferrous sulfate and tetracycline's levels. There are no clinically significant drug-to-herbal interactions established for ferrous sulfate.

9. Discuss client education for IDA. Because iron is best absorbed on an empty stomach, clients should be advised to take the supplement one hour before meals. However, if the iron supplement causes gastric distress such as nausea or heartburn, the supplement should be taken with meals. The client should comply with the medication prescription. All meals must include foods high in iron. Inform the client that if the supplement is taken with food, it decreases the absorption and takes longer to replenish

iron stores. Inform the client that the liquid forms of iron cause less gastrointestinal distress but they stain the teeth, therefore, the liquid should be taken with a straw, and the mouth should be rinsed with water after the liquid is taken. The client should avoid antacids or dairy products because they diminish the absorption of iron. Inform the client that the color of the stool may be dark green or black, and that this is normal. The client must keep appointments for evaluation of blood counts to determine if the anemia is resolving or redeveloping.

10. Explain nursing implications for clients with IDA. Nurses should be aware that older clients are more prone to IDA, mostly because of poor nutritional intake and a decreased absorption of iron. Therefore, during the initial interview, nurses should include in the assessment history, height, weight, and nutritional screening, evaluating dietary patterns for foods high in iron and assessment. The nurse should also focus on eliciting questions pertaining to her menstrual cycle to determine if abnormal bleeding may be the cause of the decrease in iron. Asking questions pertaining to gastrointestinal function such as diarrhea is important since persistent diarrhea interferes with the absorption of iron, preventing it from entering the bloodstream in the required amount, even though the dietary intake is adequate.

References

Black, J. M. and Hawks, J. H. (2005). *Medical-Surgical Nursing: Clinical Management for Positive Outcomes.* Philadelphia: W. B. Saunders.

Broyles, B. E. (2005). *Medical-Surgical Nursing Clinical Companion.* Durham, NC: Carolina Academic Press.

Corbet, J. V. (2004). *Laboratory Tests and Diagnostic Procedures with Nursing Diagnoses* (6th ed.). Upper Saddle River, NJ: Prentice Hall.

Gahart, B. L. and Nazareno, A. R. (2005). *2005 Intraveneous Medications.* St. Louis: Elsevier Mosby.

Huether, S. E. and McCance, K. L. (2004). *Understanding Pathophysiology* (3rd ed.). St. Louis: Mosby.

Ignatavicius, D. D. and Workman, M. L. (2006). *Medical-Surgical Nursing across the Health Care Continuum* (5th ed.). Philadelphia: W. B. Saunders.

Spratto, G. R. and Woods, A. L. (2005). *2005 Edition: PDR Nurse's Drug Handbook.* Clifton Park, NY: Thomson Delmar Learning.

CASE STUDY 2

Folic Acid Deficiency Anemia

GENDER

M

AGE

56

SETTING

- Clinic

ETHNICITY/CULTURE

- White American

PREEXISTING CONDITIONS

- Alcohol consumption
- Poor nutrition

COEXISTING CONDITIONS

LIFESTYLE

- Consumes only one meal per day for several years.
- Consumes three cans of beer daily

COMMUNICATION

DISABILITY

SOCIOECONOMIC STATUS

- Low

SPIRITUAL/RELIGIOUS

- Anglican

PHARMACOLOGIC

- Multivitamin
- Leucovorin calcium (Folinic acid)
- Folic acid (Apo-Folic)

PSYCHOSOCIAL

- Anxiety
- Denial

LEGAL

ETHICAL

- Do nurses have an obligation to care for clients with a lifestyle disease?
- What considerations should be made for substance abusers who are being treated for other medical problems?

ALTERNATIVE THERAPY

PRIORITIZATION

- Maintain safety of the client and others
- Observe for additional signs and symptoms of substance overdose

DELEGATION

- RN
- Detox health care provider

MODERATE

THE DIGESTIVE AND URINARY SYSTEMS

Level of difficulty: Moderate

Overview: This case involves prioritizing, using critical thinking skills, and appropriate delegation of staff to effectively care for this client. Assessment for signs of psychiatric and neurological manifestations is paramount, and safety is a major issue that must be maintained at all times.

Client Profile

Mr. W, a 56-year-old male, is brought by emergency medical service (EMS) to the hospital emergency department (ED) for the fourth time in one month. On this occasion, the client was seen wandering along a highway throwing used bottles at passing vehicles. Previous hospital medical records reveal a history of alcoholism. Mr. W lives alone in a one-bedroom apartment. He has a sister who is 74 years old but lives in another state. On admission, his chief concern is his pounding heart, which occurs frequently. His vital signs are:

> Blood pressure: 130/88
> Pulse: 104
> Respirations: 14
> Temperature: 99.4° F

Case Study

With a calm and deliberate approach, the ED nurse begins the initial interview while providing safety for the client and self. The ED nurse monitors for signs of psychiatric and neurological manifestations, and maintains safety. Physical assessment finds no injuries of Mr. W's head and there are no bruises on his body. He has a beefy red tongue, generalized weakness, and is unable to stand unassisted for even brief periods. There are tremors of both hands, and he complains of burning on the soles of his feet. There is hand and feet paresthesia and decreased perception of vibration and position. He has poor deep-tendon reflexes. There are enlarged veins noted under the skin around the navel, and his abdomen is slightly distended. The nurse practitioner (NP) in the ED continues with the assessment and makes a tentative diagnosis of folic acid deficiency anemia (FADA). She orders the following laboratory tests: serum folate levels, thiamin, total calcium, magnesium, alcohol blood levels, and urine drug test. The labs are drawn and sent for analysis. The results are:

> Folic acid: 3 ng/Ml
> Thiamin: 140 pg/mL
> Total calcium: 8 mg/dL
> Magnesium: 0.90 mEq/L
> Albumin: 2 g/dL
> Alcohol blood level: 80 mg/dL
> Urine drug test: positive for alcohol only

After a health care provider and the NP review the lab results, a diagnosis of FADA secondary to alcoholism is confirmed. The client is transferred to a medical unit for further evaluations, including ruling out alcoholic polyneuropathy and Wernicke-Korsakoff syndrome and for detoxification as needed.

Questions

1. Discuss the pathophysiology of FADA.

2. What are priority nursing interventions for the intoxicated client diagnosed with FADA upon access to the emergency department?

3. Discuss the significance of Mr. W's lab values as they relate to his diagnosis of FADA.

4. Discuss common nursing diagnoses for the intoxicated client with a diagnosis of FADA.

5. Discuss ethical issues as they relate to laboratory tests for persons assumed to consume abnormal amounts of alcohol.

6. What are the purposes for the prescribed orders?

7. What are the most common adverse reactions, drug-to-drug interactions, and drug-to-food/herbal interactions of the prescribed medications?

8. Discuss the purpose for the registered dietitian's evaluation of the client's nutritional status.

9. Discuss the role of the social worker for clients.

10. Discuss client education for FADA and alcoholism.

Questions and Suggested Answers

1. Discuss the pathophysiology of FADA. Folic acid is required for deoxyribose nucleic acid (DNA) synthesis leading to red blood cell (RBC) formation and maturation. The main metabolic consequence of folic acid deficiency is altering of DNA metabolism. This results in changes in cellular nuclear morphology, especially in those cells with the most rapid rates of multiplication: RBCs, leukocytes, and epithelial cells of the stomach, intestines, vagina, and uterine cervix.

2. What are priority nursing interventions for the intoxicated client diagnosed with FADA upon access to the ED? The nurse's priority as the client enters the ED is safety. The nurse should stay with the client as much as possible or delegate a one-to-one assignment to a nursing attendant while reality orientation remains ongoing. Because agitation and anxiety are common, the client should be assessed for increasing belligerence and the potential for violence. The nurse should inform a supervisor that this classified client is in the ED, because the client is at high risk for injury due to lack of coordination and impaired judgment. In this situation, a private room with one-to-one observation will be needed along with protective measures. Serum specimen for blood alcohol level is drawn and sent for analysis, and it is critical for the nurse to continue assessment and interventions until the blood alcohol content (BAC) has decreased to at least 100 mg/dL and until any associated disorders or injuries have been ruled out.

3. Discuss the significance of Mr. W's lab values as they relate to his diagnosis of FADA? The *serum folate level* is decreased, indicating that his nutritional intake has probably been lacking in foods such as green leafy vegetables, liver, yeast, citrus fruits, dried beans, which are the most common cause. The decrease in *thiamin* is strongly related to alcohol abuse, because alcohol interferes with the absorption and distribution of many vitamins that are found to be deficient in alcoholics. The deficiency in *calcium* and *magnesium* are related to the effects of prolonged intake of alcohol on bone marrow function. The increase in *alcohol blood level* is significant to know for the purpose of detoxification but also to evaluate risk of Wernicke-Korsakoff syndrome, which occurs as a consequence of a thiamine deficiency in predisposed persons after many years of excessive alcohol consumption. *Urine drug testing* provides help in detecting the presence of drug/alcohol consumption within a specified time frame. Urine testing is typically qualitative and notes the presence or absence of the substance.

4. Discuss common nursing diagnoses for the intoxicated client with a diagnosis of FADA?

- Risk for injury R/T sensorimotor deficits, seizure activity, and confusion – The nurse should assess for risk factors such as unsteady gait, tremors, and seizure activity and provide safety measures to prevent injury. The nurse should monitor vital signs frequently, especially heart rate, because prompt recognition will prevent progression of autonomic nervous systems symptoms that could develop.
- Disturbed sensory perception (auditory and/or visual) R/T sensory overload – The nurse should assess the client's level of orientation to reality and to determine appropriate interventions. The client will need a quiet, nonstimulating, well-lit environment to reduce external stimuli and calm an overactive central nervous system (CNS).
- Imbalanced nutrition: less than body requirements – The nurse should assess client's dietary intake, monitor food/fluid, and calculate daily caloric intake to determine if nutritional needs are being met or if modification is needed.
- Risk for self-directed violence R/T hallucinations and altered thought processes – Requires assessment of impulse control (usually poor) or panic to implement emergency management in the event the client becomes destructive; provision of a safe environment to prevent injury to self or others; implementation of chemical restraints as necessary to prevent escalation of threatening behaviors. The health care provider must use calmness along with a reassuring and consistent approach so as to benefit the client.

5. Discuss ethical issues as they relate to laboratory tests for persons assumed to consume abnormal amounts of alcohol. Ethical issues that continue to be of concern with drug testing include potential infringement of civil rights and the issue of obtaining the client's informed consent; a large number of variables may affect the results, and shortcomings of urine samples include privacy issues surrounding the sample collection and possibilities of sample dilution/substitution or alteration by deceptive clients.

The following are prescribed:

- Intravenous fluid 5% dextrose in water (D5%W) with 5 mL multiple vitamin at 125 mL/hr
- Leucovorin calcium (Folinic acid) 1 mg IV × 24 hours
- Folic acid (Apo-Folic) 0.4 mg daily
- Have registered dietitian see the client
- Have the social worker see the client

6. What are the purposes for the prescribed orders? The *intravenous fluid* replenishes insensible loss and rehydrates the client. The *multivitamin* replenishes needed vitamins that are the daily requirement of a balanced nutrition that has not been replenished due to inadequate nutritional intake. *Leucovorin calcium* intravenously ensures a rapid response to the stimulation of the production of RBCs, white blood cells (WBCs), and platelets in clients with megaloblastic anemias. It improves symptoms of glossitis, weight loss, fatigue, restless legs, irritability, muscular pain, mental depression, and forgetfulness. *Folic acid* stimulates the production of RBCs, WBCs, and platelets in clients with megaloblastic anemia such as FADA. *Folic acid* is prescribed for daily intake because the deficiency is more related to poor nutritional intake and must be corrected by dietary measures, which includes folic acid, a vitamin.

7. What are the most common adverse reactions, drug-to-drug interactions, and drug-to-food/herbal interactions of the prescribed medications? Common adverse reactions, drug-to-drug, drug-to-food/herbal interactions of *multivitamin* are not clinically established. The most common adverse reactions of *leucovorin calcium* are allergic reaction and rash. Drug-to-drug interactions may occur with the simultaneous use of barbiturates, phenytoin, or primidone, which may decrease anticonvulsant effect. High doses contain significant alcohol and may cause increased CNS depression when used with CNS depressants. Simultaneous use with trimethoprim/sulfamethoxazole may decrease result in anti-ineffective efficacy and poor therapeutic outcome when used to treat pneumocystis carinii pneumonia in HIV clients. The simultaneous use with fluorouracil increases fluorouracil therapeutic and toxic effects. There are no clinically significant drug-to-food/herbal interactions established. The most common adverse reactions of *folic acid* are allergic reaction and rash. Drug-to-drug interactions may occur with the simultaneous use of pyrimethamine, methotrexate, trimethoprim, and triamterene, which may prevent the activation of folic acid. The simultaneous use with sulfonamides including sulfasalazine, antacids, and cholestyramine decreases the absorption of folic acid. Estrogens, phenytoin, phenobarbital, primidone, carbamazepine, or corticosteroids when used simultaneously with folic acid increase the requirements of folic acid.

8. Discuss the purpose for the registered dietitian's evaluation of the client's nutritional status. A registered dietitian is needed to evaluate the client's nutritional states and provide recommendations and sample meal plans to health care providers involved in the client's plan of care. Assessment of the client's nutritional status involves measuring both the degree to which the physiological need for nutrients is being met and the degree of balance between nutrient intake and nutrient expenditure. The components of a nutritional assessment that is included in the registered dietitian's assessment include the health history, diet history, evaluation of food intake, and physical examination.

9. Discuss the role of the social worker for clients. The social worker facilitates appropriate client discharge and follow-up care to ensure proper use of community services. The social worker assigned to Mr. W's case may seek placement in a residential setting where the client can be more frequently supervised after discharge.

10. Discuss client education for FADA and alcoholism. Develop a trusting relationship with the client, then attempt to have client verbalize constructive coping mechanisms and strategies he will use upon discharge to prevent injury to himself and others, or complications of the disease that could occur. Emphasize to the client the importance of complying with medication instructions, and to not exceed the prescribed dose of folic acid. Stress the importance of maintaining balanced diet, including foods high in folic acid; discuss the importance of the diet with the client. Inform the client that although FADA can develop because of several causes, the most commonly cited cause is alcoholism. Emphasize the negative effects of alcohol on all body systems and the serious complications that usually develop over time.

References

Black, J. M., Hawks, J. H., and Keene, A. M. (2005). *Medical-Surgical Nursing* (7th ed.). Philadelphia: W. B. Saunders.

Broyles, B. E. (2005). *Medical-Surgical Nursing Clinical Companion*. Durham, NC: Carolina Academic Press.

"Folic Acid." www.rxmed.com.

Fortinsah, K. M. and Holoday-Worret. P. A. (2004). *Psychiatric Mental Health Nursing* (3rd ed.). St. Louis: Mosby.

Gahart, B. L. and Nazareno, A. R. (2005). *2005 Intravenous Medications*. St. Louis: Mosby.

Huether, S. E. and McCance, K. L. (2004). *Understanding Pathophysiology* (3rd ed.). St. Louis: Mosby.

Ignatavicius, D. D. and Workman, M. L. (2006). *Medical-Surgical Nursing: Critical Thinking for Collaborative Care* (5th ed.). Philadelphia: W. B. Saunders.

Spratto, G. R. and Woods, A. L. (2005). *2005 Edition: PDR Nurse's Drug Handbook*. Clifton Park, NY: Thomson Delmar Learning.

Symptomatic Cholelithiasis/Cholecystectomy

GENDER	**SPIRITUAL/RELIGIOUS**
F	■ Evangelical
AGE	**PHARMACOLOGIC**
45	■ Morphine sulfate (Duramorph)
SETTING	■ Lorazepam (Ativan)
■ Hospital	■ Ampicillin sodium (Omnipen-N)
	■ Ursodiol (Actigall)
ETHNICITY/CULTURE	■ Midazolam HcL (Versed)
■ Native American	**PSYCHOSOCIAL**
PREEXISTING CONDITIONS	■ Anxiety
■ Diabetes mellitus type 1	■ Pain
COEXISTING CONDITIONS	**LEGAL**
■ Obesity	**ETHICAL**
LIFESTYLE	**ALTERNATIVE THERAPY**
■ Restaurant cashier	■ Meditation
COMMUNICATION	**PRIORITIZATION**
	■ Assess & relieve pain
DISABILITY	■ Prepare client for diagnostic testing
	DELEGATION
SOCIOECONOMIC STATUS	■ RN
■ Low	■ CNA
	■ Client education

M O D E R A T E

THE DIGESTIVE AND URINARY SYSTEMS

Level of difficulty: Moderate

Overview: This case involves thorough history and physical exam to achieve accurate diagnosis, because biliary colic and coronary artery disease have similar symptoms, and a diagnosis is often tentatively made based on symptoms alone. Careful assessment of the skin for jaundice helps to determine cause of symptoms. The nurse should be able to prioritize and delegate with a mixed group of clients requesting nursing interventions simultaneously. The certified nursing assistant (CNA) can obtain height, weight, and vital signs.

Client Profile

Ms. C is a 45-year-old client who is admitted via the emergency department (ED) to the surgical unit with complaints of vague pain at the right upper quadrant of her body, which has gotten more noticeable after she had a meal that was high in fatty foods. Ms. C is 5'4" and weighs 205 pounds.

Case Study

Further interviewing reveals Ms. C's past medical history (PMH) includes Type I diabetes, the use of birth control pills for 15 years, history of cholelithiasis that was previously treated with ursodiol, and a family history of gallstones. Her vital signs are:

Blood pressure: 120/78
Pulse: 78
Respirations: 20
Temperature: 100.4° F

During this portion of the interview, Ms. C explains that the pain is getting worse, especially in the right upper abdominal quadrant, and is presently radiating to the back at the right shoulder area. As she explains, she is moving about in the chair and states she now feels nauseous and wants to vomit. She retches on few occasions, but does not vomit. After a while, the triage nurse continues with the physical assessment, and on light palpation of the abdomen, the nurse finds marked tenderness of the right upper quadrant when Ms. C is asked to breath in deeply. Ms. C is now complaining of spasms of the abdomen. The health care provider is immediately notified, arrives, and assesses the client. Morphine sulfate IM stat and lorazepam (Ativan) 4 mg IM are administered as ordered with effective outcome as verbalized by Ms. C 25 minutes after the medication was administered. Additional information pertaining to her medical and surgical history is gathered by the health care provider, who makes a tentative diagnosis of acute cholelithiasis. A chest X-ray and EKG are done and reveal normal findings. An abdominal X-ray finds calcified gallstones, and upper gastrointestinal (GI) radiographic series is negative for gastritis or peptic ulcers. Serum labs are drawn and sent to the lab. The results are:

Aspartate aminotransferase (AST): 40 u/L
Alakine phosphatase (ALP): 118 u/L
LDH_4 and LDH_5: 15%
Prothrombin time (PT): 18.9 (Ref. 10.4 –15.3)
Partial thromboplastin time (PTT): 40.5
Total bilirubin: 1.4

Platelet count (PLT): 150,000/mm^3
Hematocrit (Hct): 30.4%
Hemoglobin (Hgb): 11 g/mL
Direct bilirubin: 1.1 mg/dL

Ms. C is sent for an ultrasonography, which identifies gallstones in the common bile duct and gallbladder. Upon return from the procedure, the health care provider discusses the findings of the diagnostic studies and the plan of care with Ms. C, which includes a lithotripsy and possibly a laparoscopic cholecystectomy. After she is allowed quality time to asked questions, and receive answers, an informed consent is explained by the health care provider. Ms. C signs the consent for both the lithotripsy and the cholecystectomy.

Questions

1. Discuss the incidence and prevalence of gallstones' occurrence in the United States.

2. Discuss women's considerations for gallstone formation.

3. Discuss some of the contributing risk factors of cholelithiasis (gallstones).

4. If gallstones are lodged within the gall bladder or cystic duct, tissue spasm occurs in an effort to mobilize the stone. Discuss the clinical symptoms the client may manifest at this time.

5. What are some common nursing diagnoses for the client with gallstone disease?

6. What are the most common adverse reactions, drug-to-drug interactions, and drug-to-food/herbal interactions for the prescribed medications?

7. What are the purposes for the prescribed orders including *ursodeoxycholic acid*?

8. Discuss various procedures for the removal of gallstones.

9. Discuss client education post-cholecystectomy.

Questions and Suggested Answers

1. Discuss the incidence and prevalence of gallstones' occurrence in the United States. More than 20 million persons in the United States have gallbladder disease, resulting in over 800,000 hospitalizations per year. It is more commonly seen in persons over 40 years of age, and women account for 70% of the cases. Native Americans and American Indians, particularly the Pima Indians of Arizona, have an unusually high incidence of gallstones, with Mexican Americans and white American individuals following. Cholesterol calculi are the most common form of gallstones found in the

United States, accounting for 90% of all gallstones. They generally originate from the gallbladder.

2. **Discuss women's considerations for gallstone formation.** Women who
are between 20 and 60 years of age are twice as likely as men to develop
gallstones. Obesity is a major risk factor for gallstone formation, especially
in women. Pregnancy leads to worsened gallstone formation. Pregnancy, as
well as drugs such as estrogen and birth control pills, especially the older
oral contraceptives, alter hormone levels and delay muscular contraction
of the gallbladder, causing a decreased rate of bile emptying. The incidence is higher in women who have had multiple pregnancies.

3. **Discuss some of the contributing risk factors of cholelithiasis (gallstones).** The actual cause of gallstones is unknown. However, cholelithiasis
develops when the balance that keeps cholesterol, bile salts, and calcium in
solution is altered so that precipitation of these substances occurs. Gallstones
may also develop when the client with cholelithiasis secretes bile from the
liver. The bile may be supersaturated with cholesterol (have more than the
required amount of cholesterol), resulting in precipitation of cholesterol
stones. The precipitation of "microstones" results in aggregation of more
crystals, which grow to form "macrostones." This process usually occurs in
the gallbladder, because the gallbladder has decreased motility. Stones may
even accumulate and fill the entire gallbladder. The changes in the composition of bile are also significant in the formation of gallstones. This occurs
when stasis of bile leads to progression of the supersaturation and changes in
the chemical composition of bile, resulting in the development of gallstones.
Drugs such as gemfibrozil (Lopid) increases biliary cholesterol saturation
and, in so doing, increases the risk of gallstones formation.

4. **If gallstones are lodged within the gall bladder or cystic duct, tissue
spasm occurs in an effort to mobilize the stone. Discuss the clinical symptoms the client may manifest at this time.** *Pain* as the stones migrate to the
cystic duct or to the common bile duct. *Obstructive jaundice*, because there
is no bile flow into the duodenum. *Dark amber urine,* which foams when
shaken, because soluble bilirubin is in the urine. The **urine is negative for
urobilinogen**, because there is no bilirubin reaching the small intestine to
be converted to urobilinogen. Clay-colored stools, because there is no
bilirubin reaching the small intestine to be converted to urobilinogen.
Pruritus, due to the deposition of bile salts in the skin tissues. *Intolerance to
fatty foods* (nausea, sensation of fullness, anorexia), because there is no bile
in the small intestine for fat digestion. *Bleeding tendencies*, because of lack
of or decreased absorption of vitamin K, resulting in decreased production
of prothrombin. *Steatorrhea*, because there are no bile salts in the duodenum, preventing fat emulsion and digestion.

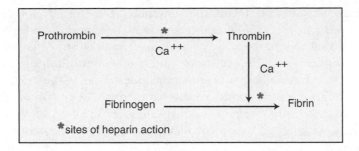

Gallstones can block the outflow of bile from the gallbladder.

5. What are some common nursing diagnoses for the client with gallstone disease?

- Pain R/T biliary spasms
- Risk for deficient fluid volume R/T vomiting and nasogastric suctioning
- Anxiety R/T pain and potential for lithotripsy or surgery
- Deficient knowledge R/T condition, treatment, and health maintenance

The following are prescribed in preparation for laparoscopic cholecystectomy:

- Keep NPO. Start IV line with 0.9% normal saline at 125 mLs per hour
- Morphine sulfate (Duramorph) 1–2 mg IV q1–2h PRN for pain
- Lorazepam (Ativan) 0.5 mg IV q4h PRN for nausea
- Ampicillin sodium (Omnipen-N) 1 g IV on call to the OR
- Midazolam HcL (Versed) 2.5 mg IV on call to OR

6. What are the most common adverse reactions, drug-to-drug, drug-to-food/herbal interactions for the prescribed medications? The most common adverse effects associated with *intravenous infusion of 0.9% sodium chloride* is hypernatremia and fluid retention. These effects depend on how rapidly the infusion is administered and other health alterations the client may have. The most common adverse reactions with intravenous *morphine sulfate* include drowsiness, disturbances in gait risking falls, sleepiness, and constipation. Respiratory effects are dose-related and occur infrequently. The most common adverse effects of intravenous *lorazepam* include drowsiness, hypotension, hallucinations, restlessness, and a risk of respiratory depression that is dose-related. The most common adverse reactions of *ampicillin sodium* are hypersensitivity responses, diarrhea, and superinfections, although diarrhea and superinfections are unlikely with a single dose.

The only drug-to-drug interaction that may occur with *intravenous sodium chloride* is mannitol, which can result in severe phlebitis at the site of infusion, if administered together. With intravenous *morphine sulfate*, drug-to-drug interactions may occur with the simultaneous use of alcohol, other central nervous system (CNS) depressants, general anesthesia, antidepressants, barbiturates, hypnotics, sedatives, histamine-2 antagonists, and chlorpromazine that will increase CNS depression and possibly result in respiratory depression. Morphine sulfate may antagonize the effects of metoclopramide, and anticholinergics and antidiarrheals may increase the risk of constipation, and when used with diuretics, antihypertensive agents, ganglionic blocking agents, antidepressants, benzodiazepines, adrenergic blockers, calcium channel blockers, calcium, nitroprusside sodium, and nitroglycerin, hypotensive risks are increased. Concurrent use with rifampin may decrease morphine's analgesic effects, and extended respiratory depression or prolonged blockade with neuromuscular blocking agents may occur when used with morphine (Gahart and Nazareno, 820).

Drug-to-drug interactions may occur with the simultaneous use of intravenous *lorazepam* and alcohol, antihistamines, barbiturates, MAO inhibitors, opioid analgesics, phenothiazines, and tricyclic antidepressants, which will increase CNS depression. Concurrent administration with valproate or probenicid will increase the effects of lorazepam by decreasing its clearance. "Apnea, bradycardia, cardiac arrest, and coma have been reported when used concurrently with haloperidol" (Gahart and Nazareno, 741). Although rare, significant hypotension, respiratory depression, and stupor have occurred with the simultaneous use of loxapine. *Lorazepam* may increase the serum levels of digoxin and phenytoin and, as with other drugs in its class, lorazepam may increase the risk of zidovudine toxicity. Theophyllines and estrogen-containing oral contraceptives decrease the effects of lorazepam. If used in conjunction with scopolamine, there is an increased risk of sedation, hallucinations, and confused behavior.

Drug-to-drug interactions may occur with the simultaneous use of *intravenous ampicillin sodium* and allopurinol, which increases the incidence of rash. Streptomycin potentiates the bactericidal effects ampicillin has against enterococci. Although they may be used concurrently with aminoglycosides, they should never be mixed in the same infusion due to altering of the action of gentamycin. Use with beta-adrenergic blocking agents may increase the risk of anaphylaxis and decrease ampicillin's effectiveness.

Ampicillin sodium is potentiated by probenecid, and ampicillin decreases the effectiveness of oral contraceptives. There is an increased risk of bleeding when used concurrently with heparin.

No clinically significant drug-to-food/herbal interactions are established. Drug-to-drug interactions may occur with the simultaneous use of intravenous *midazolam HcL* and alcohol, CNS depressants, inhalation anesthetics, opiod analgesics phenothiazines, thiopental, tricyclic antidepressants, and anticonvulsants, which may potentiate CNS depression. Azole antifungals, cimetidine, diltiazem, verapamil, macrolide antibiotics, omeprazole, and ranitidine decrease the clearance of IV midazolam, thus increasing its effects. Protease inhibitors may increase risk of prolonged sedation. Use with ritonavir is contraindicated because of the high risk of life-threatening sedation and respiratory depression (Gahart and Nazareno, 803). Midazolam may potentiate the action of digoxin and increase the hypotensive effects of benzodiazepines. Concurrent use with rifampin or theophylline decreases the effects of benzodiazepines including midazolam. Smoking decreases serum levels of midazolam, thus decreasing its effectiveness. There are no clinically significant drug-to-food interactions established for intravenous midazolam, however, grapefruit juice decreases the absorption and simultaneous use of kava-kava and valerian may potentiate sedating effects.

7. What are the purposes for the prescribed orders including *ursodeoxycholic acid*? *Nothing by mouth (NPO)* is prescribed to prevent nausea and vomiting (and risk of aspiration) prior to anesthesia. The *0.9% normal saline* (an isotonic fluid) *infusion* maintains fluid hydration, expands intravascular volume, and provides readiness for blood transfusion if needed. *Morphine sulfate* is a Schedule II opioid analgesic, relieves pain by binding with the same receptors and endogenous opioid peptides, resulting in euphoria, and analgesia at the spinal level. *Lorazepam* is a benzodiazepine antianxiety agent that also is an effective antiemetic through its depressive effects on the emetic center of the CNS and relaxes the smooth muscle of the gallbladder, which helps to decrease gall bladder spasm. *Ampicillin sodium* is a broad-spectrum antibiotic that is highly bactericidal even at low concentrations. It is used for this client as prophylaxis prior to surgery to prevent infection. Since the abdomen is an area of the body that will also be incised during the procedure, ampicillin, a broad-spectrum antibiotic, is administered to destroy both gram-positive and gram-negative organisms, which can invade the procedural site, causing postprocedural infection. It functions to retard the infectious process with its highly bactericidal action that inhibits protein synthesis, destroying organisms. *Midazolam HcL* is a commonly used short-acting benzodiazepine CNS depressant on call to the OR. Further, it has an amnesic effect. These effects occur due to midazolam's binding to specific receptor binding sites in the brain, resulting in production of anxiolytic effects, sedation, and muscle relaxation.

8. Discuss various procedures for the removal of gallstones. There are two nonsurgical approaches for biliary stone removal. Most clients are treated by means of endoscopic retrograde cholangiopancreatography (ERCP). Standard ERCP techniques will clear stones from the biliary tree in approximately 90% of the clients. ERCP allows for visualization of the biliary system, as well as the placement of stents and sphincterotomy (papillotomy) if warranted.

Endoscopic sphincterotomy is especially effective in removing common bile duct stones. The endoscope is passed to the duodenum. An electro-diathermy knife is attached to the endoscope, which is used to make an incision on the sphincter muscle to widen the sphincter of Oddi. A basket is used to retrieve the stone, or the stone may be left in the duodenum and will be passed out naturally in the stool. If the stone is too large to pass through the duct, the endoscopist can crush the stone (mechanical lithotripsy). However, this mechanical lithotripsy can cause ERCP-induced acute pancreatitis.

The extracorpeal shock-wave lithotripsy (ESWL) uses high-energy shock waves to disintegrate the gallstones. For this procedure, the client must have a functioning gallbladder. An ultrasound scan is first done to locate the stones and to determine where to direct the shock waves. The shock waves are directed through the abdomen as a water-filled cushion is pressed against the area. The procedure usually takes one to two hours to disintegrate the stones. After they are broken up, the fragments pass through the common bile duct and into the small intestine.

Laparoscopic cholecystectomy is the treatment of choice for cholecystectomy. Currently, approximately 92% of all cholecystomies are performed laparoscopically. In this procedure, the gallbladder is removed through one of four small punctures in the abdomen. A one-centimeter puncture is made slightly above the umbilicus, and the surgeon inflates the abdominal cavity with three to four liters of CO_2, to improve visibility. The laparoscope, which has a camera attached to it, is inserted into the abdomen. Two additional punctures are made just below the ribs, one on the right anterior axillary line and the other on the right midclavicular line. These punctures are used for insertion of grasping forceps. A dissection laser is inserted into the fourth puncture, which is made just right of the midsection.

Using closed-circuit monitors to view the abdominal cavity, the surgeon retracts and dissects the gallbladder and removes it with grasping forceps. Advantages of the laparoscopic cholecystectomy include decreased postoperative pain, shorter hospital stay and earlier return to work. The main complication is injury to the common bile duct. Contraindications to laparoscopic cholecystectomy are peritonitis, cholangitis, gangrene or perforation of the gallbladder, portal hypertension, and serious bleeding disorders.

9. Discuss client education post-cholecystectomy. The client should be instructed to remove the bandages on the puncture site upon returning home, and may bathe or shower. Emphasize the need to report redness, swelling, or bile-colored drainage or pus from any of the incisions. The client is informed to report severe abdominal pain, nausea, vomiting, fever, and chills. The client should resume normal activities gradually and can return to work in one week from the day of surgery. The client can resume a normal diet unless otherwise directed by the surgeon.

References

Broyles, B. E. (2005). *Medical-Surgical Nursing Clinical Companion*. Durham, NC: Carolina Academic Press.

Corbet, J. V. (2004). *Laboratory Tests and Diagnostic Procedures with Nursing Diagnoses* (6th ed.). Upper Saddle River, NJ: Prentice Hall.

Deglin, J. H. and Vallerand, A. H. (2005). *Davis's Drug Guide for Nurses* (9th ed.). Philadelphia: F. A. Davis.

Gahart, B. L. and Nazareno, A. R. (2005). *2005 Intravenous Medications*. St. Louis: Mosby.

Huether, S. E. and McCance, K. L. (2004). *Understanding Pathophysiology* (3rd ed.). St. Louis: Mosby.

Ignatavicius, D. D. and Workman, M. L. (2006). *Medical-Surgical Nursing across the Health Care Continuum*. (5th ed.). Philadelphia: W. B. Saunders.

Lewis, S. M., McLean Heitkemper, M., and Dirksen, S. R. (2004). *Medical-Surgical Nursing: Assessment and Management of Clinical Problems* (6th ed.). St. Louis: Mosby.

Paul, M. G., McGuire, A. M., Burris, D. G., and Thorfinnson, E. D. (2005) "New Techniques in the Management of Common Bile Duct Sstones." Available at www.foxhall.com.

Spratto, G. R. and Woods, A. L. (2005). *2005 Edition: PDR Nurse's Drug Handbook*. Clifton Park, NY: Thomson Delmar Learning.

CASE STUDY 4

Laennec's (Alcoholic) Cirrhosis

GENDER

M

AGE

60

SETTING

■ Hospital

ETHNICITY/CULTURE

■ White American

PREEXISTING CONDITIONS

COEXISTING CONDITIONS

■ Alcoholic liver disease

LIFESTYLE

■ Unemployed
■ Previously employed by fire department

COMMUNICATION

DISABILITY

■ Inability to perform moderate amount of activity of daily living (ADL)

SOCIOECONOMIC STATUS

■ Low

SPIRITUAL/RELIGION

■ Catholic

PHARMACOLOGIC

■ Spironolactone (Aldactone)
■ Malgaldrate (Riopan)
■ Thiamine
■ Folic acid (Apo-Folic)
■ Magnesium
■ Sulfate
■ Phytonadione (Aqua-Mephyton)
■ Neomycin sulfate (Mycifradin sulfate)
■ Propranolol HcL (Inderal)
■ Hydrochlorothiazide (HydroDIURIL)

PSYCHOSOCIAL

■ Anxicty
■ Fear
■ Agitation
■ Depression
■ Emotional liability

LEGAL

ETHICAL

■ Alcoholism is a disease. The client has a right to quality care. Health care providers, though they may not approve of alcohol abuse, have a responsibility to assist in the care of these persons in need.

ALTERNATIVE THERAPY

PRIORITIZATION

■ Monitor level of orientation
■ Administer medications as prescribed

DELEGATION

■ RN   ■   CNA

THE DIGESTIVE AND URINARY SYSTEMS

Level of difficulty: Difficult

Overview: This case will involve critical thinking skills to appropriately delegate assignment to competent health care personnel who are skilled in identifying potential indicators for pending complications, and who are able to function independently in an emergency setting such as a busy emergency department. The case involves caring for clients with bleeding esophageal varices, requiring balloon tamponade. Assign certified nursing attendant to remain with the client on a 1:1 schedule as needed.

DIFFICULT

Client Profile

Mr. S is a 60-year-old male with history of alcohol cirrhosis and ascites. Mr. S has had multiple re-admissions for severel paracentesis. He was recently read-mitted to the hospital for ventral hernia following a repair for protrusion of the umbilical tissue. Mr. S is 5'8" and weighs 194 pounds.

Case Study

Mr. S is seen in the outpatient clinic of the hospital by referral from a neighborhood community health care center. A nurse practitioner (NP) initiates the interview. Mr. S is alert and oriented to time place and person, but complains of being unusually tired after minimum exercise such as walking four short blocks. His vital signs:

Blood pressure: 140/70
Pulse: 76
Respirations: 20
Temperature: 100.4° F

His lungs are clear, his abdomen is distended with decreased bowel sounds at all quadrants. On palpation, his liver is large and firm with a sharp edge. He reports frequent episodes of anorexia, frequent indigestion, and con-stipation alternating with diarrhea. His social history includes frequent alcohol intake and history of intoxication during his employment, espe-cially on weekends. He reports living with his younger sister for several years, but he has been living by himself in a one-bedroom apartment. He reports losing his job because of the "frequent delays of his mode of trans-portation" he uses for his commute to work. He is "not in contact with his parents for several years" and did not provide name/s of significant others.

After the history and physical assessment was completed, the nurse prac-titioner (NP) made a tentative diagnosis of Laennec's cirrhosis pending additional labs, diagnostic tests, and review of data by a multidisciplinary team. Mr. S's laboratory values are:

Glucose: 118 mg/dL
Total leukocyte count: 9,000 cell/mm^3
Hematocrit (Hct): 36%
Activated coagulation time: 130 seconds
Prothrombin time (PT) with INR: 4
Partial thromboplastin time (PTT): 80 seconds
Total bilirubin: 1.6 mg/dl
Direct bilirubin: 0.9 mg/dl
Indirect bilirubin: 1.4 mg/dl

Alkaline-phosphate: 272 U/L

Serum glutamic-oxaloacetic transaminase (SGOT or aspartate transaminase): 44 U/L

Serum glutamic-pyrevic transaminase (SGPT or alanine transaminase): 48 U/L

Serum albumin: 2 g/dl

Serum globulin: 5.8 g/L

Blood urea nitrogen (BUN): 18 mg/dL

Creatinine: 2.8 mg/dl

Platelet count: 100,000/mm^3

Sodium (Na): 130 mEq/L

Potassium (K+): 3.8 mEq/L

Total calcium: 9 mg/dl

Magnesium: 1 mg/dL

Ammonia: 105 ug/dL

Daily serum labs will be monitored because the X-ray (plain) of the abdomen shows hepatomegaly and splenomegaly. Ultrasound is conclusive for portal vein thrombosis, but an esophagogastro-duodenoscopy is negative for bleeding or oozing esophageal varices, with positive gastric stomach irritation but no gastric ulceration. After the multidisciplinary team reviews all data, a diagnosis of Laennec's cirrhosis is confirmed, and the client is informed of the diagnosis and treatment plan.

Questions

1. What is your understanding of the above situation?

2. Discuss the early signs of liver cirrhosis.

3. Identify specific psychosocial findings in clients with hepatic cirrhosis.

4. Why are the total serum protein and albumin levels decreased and the prothrombin time prolonged?

5. What are the most common nursing diagnoses for cirrhosis of the liver?

6. What are the purposes for the prescribed orders?

7. What are the most common adverse reactions of the prescribed medications?

8. Discuss the drug-to-drug, drug-to-food/herbal interactions for the prescribed medications.

9. Discuss alternative invasive procedures that may be implemented if drug therapy fails to control presenting symptoms of cirrhosis of the liver.

10. If Mr. S develops massive hemorrhage and replacement blood products are not readily available, what alternatives would the health care provider prescribe?

11. If Mr. S develops portal systemic encephalopathy (PSE), what would be the probable treatment plan?

12. Discuss client education for cirrhosis of the liver.

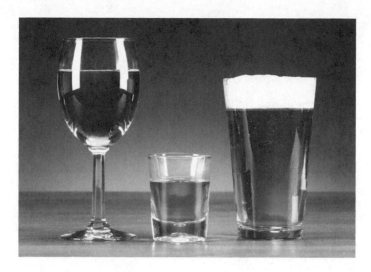

Three-fourths of cirrhosis is caused by excessive alcohol consumption.

Questions and Suggested Answers

1. **What is your understanding of the above situation?** Mr. S has developed cirrhosis of the liver due to his long history of alcohol intake. One of the most common causes for cirrhosis in the United States is alcoholic liver disease. Alcohol has a direct toxic effect on the hepatocytes and causes liver inflammation (alcoholic hepatitis). The liver becomes enlarged, with cellular degeneration and infiltration by fat, leukocytes, and lymphocytes. Over a period of time, the inflammatory process decreases and the destructive phase increases. Damage to liver tissue progresses as a result of malnutrition and repeated exposure to the alcohol. The amount of alcohol necessary to cause cirrhosis varies widely from person to person. Mr. S's history reveals frequent alcohol intake, and diagnostic studies reveal the effects of alcohol on his liver, resulting in the confirmed diagnosis.

2. **Discuss the early signs of liver cirrhosis.**

   • Anorexia, dyspepsia, flatulence, nausea and vomiting, and change in bowel habits such as diarrhea or constipation as a result of the liver's altered metabolism of carbohydrates, fats, and proteins.

   • Abdominal pain that is dull and feeling of heaviness in the right upper quadrant, due to swelling and stretching of the liver capsule, spasm of the biliary ducts, and intermittent vascular spasm.

   • Enlargement of the liver that is palpable is due to vascular changes resulting in scars and lumps.

3. **Identify specific psychosocial findings in clients with hepatic cirrhosis.**
Specific psychosocial findings in clients with hepatic cirrhosis are subtle or
obvious personality, cognitive, and behavior changes such as agitation and
belligerence and signs of emotional liability, euphoria, or depression,
which are signs and symptoms of hepatic encephalopathy. These signs and
symptoms are due to the accumulation of neurotoxins in the blood. A specific neurotoxin is ammonia, a by-product of protein metabolism.
Normally, ammonia is converted by the liver to urea before entering the
general circulation. As functional liver tissue is destroyed, ammonia can no
longer be converted to urea and it accumulates in the blood, manifesting
signs and symptoms of hepatic encephalopathy.

4. **Why are the total serum protein and albumin levels decreased and the
prothrombin time prolonged?** The serum protein and albumin levels are
decreased because one of the functions of the liver is the production of
proteins. When the liver is impaired, proteins are decreased. The prothrombin time (PT/INR) is prolonged because of the impaired production of coagulation proteins and a lack of vitamin K.

5. **What are the most common nursing diagnoses for cirrhosis of the liver?**

- Imbalanced nutrition: less than body requirements R/T anorexia,
  impaired use and storage of nutrients, nausea, and loss of nutrients
  from vomiting
- Impaired skin integrity R/T edema, ascites, and pruritus
- Ineffective breathing pattern R/T diminished sensory perception
- Risk for infection R/T leukopenia and increased susceptibility to
  environmental pathogens

The following are prescribed:

- IV infusion 0.9% NaCL 250 mL with 50 mg thiamine, folic acid 1 mg,
  5 mL multivitamin × 1
- Spironolactone (Aldactone) 100 mg PO daily
- Magaldrate (Riopan) 15 mL PO four times per day
- Thiamine (vitamin B_1) 30 mg PO daily after IV infusion is
  discontinued
- Folic acid (Apo-Folic) 1 mg PO daily after IV infusion is discontinued
- Hydrochlorothiazide (HydroDIURIL) 50 mg PO daily
- Phytonadine (Aqua-Mephyton) 120 mcg SC daily
- Diphenhydramine 25 mg PO three times per day for itching of nausea
- Repeat serum sodium level 1 hour after the infusion of 250 mL of
  NaCL IV fluid
- Daily serum labs: AST, ALT, LDH, alkaline phosphatase, total serum
  protein and albumin levels, PT/INR, PTT, platelet count, Hct, Hgb,
  sodium, potassium, blood urea nitrogen, and creatinine

6. What are the purposes for the prescribed orders? *Intravenous solution 0.9% NaCL* 250 mL with *thiamine* and *folic acid* are administered because clients with cirrhosis are malnourished and have multiple dietary deficiencies. Vitamin supplements such as thiamine, folate, and multivitamin preparations are typically added to the IV fluids because of the inability of the liver to store vitamins, and therefore, depleted stores need replacement. When IV fluid administration is discontinued, oral vitamin supplements are given. *Normal saline 0.9%* is used because the client's serum sodium level is 130 mEq/L. Repeating the serum sodium level in one hour is to determine if a higher volume of 0.9% sodium is needed to increase the sodium level.

Spironolactone is a potassium sparing diuretic that blocks aldosterone to help reduce ascites by competing with aldosterone for cellular receptor sites in the distal renal tubule and promotes sodium and chloride excretion. It prevents cardiac and respiratory discomfort caused by the pressure of ascites. It spares potassium and helps to increase the present level of serum potassium. *Riopan* is prescribed because the person with cirrhosis usually experiences frequent indigestion. Antacids such as *riopan* help to neutralize stomach acid and decrease destruction of the gut wall. *Riopan* also is beneficial because it is low in sodium content and would not contribute to the hypertension or cardiac alterations. Oral *thiamine* and *folic acid* are administered after IV therapy is discontinued to continue with the maintenance of their deficiencies. Folic acid is essential for the formation of both red and white blood cells in the bone marrow and for their maturation, which is impaired in cirrhotic states.

Hydrochlorothiazide is a thiazide diuretic that provides diuresis by acting directly on the distal convoluted tubules, promoting water excretion. *Vitamin K_1* is a fat-soluble vitamin that is given prophylactically or to correct clotting abnormalities that usually occur with cirrhotic disease. *Vitamin K_1* is essential for hepatic biosynthesis of blood clotting factors II, VII, IX, and X, and promotes liver synthesis of clotting factors. *Diphenhydramine* is an antihistamine given to help alleviate pruritus that usually occurs in clients with cirrhosis.

Daily serum labs are done because AST, ALT, and LDH may be elevated because these enzymes are released into the blood during hepatic inflammation. Alkaline phosphatase levels are sensitive to mild extrahepatic or intrahepatic biliary obstruction and therefore may increase in clients with cirrhosis. Total serum bilirubin and indirect bilirubin may rise because if the liver has begun to fail, it will not effectively excrete bilirubin. Total serum protein and albumin levels may decrease if the liver is failing, and PT/INR and PTT will be prolonged with a failing liver because of the inability of the liver to synthesize prothrombin. The platelet count is decreased, and anemia may be present with evidence of decreased Hct and

Hgb. Serum sodium and potassium are low on admission, and BUN and creatinine are borderline high and need to be monitored to prevent complications.

7. **What are the most common adverse reactions of the prescribed medications?** The most common adverse reactions of *spironolactone* are hyperkalemia, cardiac dysrhythmias, and peripheral neuropathy. The most common adverse reaction of *riopan* is constipation. There are no clinically significant adverse reactions, drug-to-drug or drug-to-food/herbal interactions, for *thiamine (Vitamin B$_1$)* established. The most common adverse reactions of *folic acid* are slight flushing and feeling of warmth when administered intravenously. The most common adverse reactions of *hydrochlorothiazide* are hypokalemia, hyperglycemia, and hyperuricemia. The most common adverse effects associated with parenteral *phytonadine* include transient flushing of the face, sweating, and weakness. The most common adverse reactions of *diphenhydramine HcL* are drowsiness, tachycardia, urinary retention, and dizziness.

8. **Discuss the drug-to-drug and drug-to-food/herbal interactions of the prescribed medications.** Drug-to-drug interactions may occur with the simultaneous use of *spironolactone* and angiotensin-converting enzymes (ACE) inhibitors, captopril, potassium salts, and triamterene, which may increase the serum potassium levels and increase toxicity and fatal dysrhythmias. When used with general anesthetics and antihypertensives, spironolactone may increase the risk of hypotension. Simultaneous use with digoxin or norepinephrine decreases the effects of these agents. Spironolactone frequently is used in conjunction with thiazide or loop diuretics to balance the potassium loss and potassium sparing. Because the naturetic effects of spironolactone are mild, it is usually prescribed in conjunction with thiazides or loop diuretics. Because aldosterone secretions are increased in congestive heart failure (CHF), this promotes body loss of potassium. Spironolactone functions to block the production of aldosterone and, in doing so, helps to prevent the excess loss of potassium. Drug-to-food interactions may occur with the use of salt substitutes and increase the risk of hyperkalemia. There are no clinically significant drug-to-herbal interactions established for spironolactone. With *riopan,* drug-to-drug interactions may occur with the simultaneous use of tetracycline because *riopan* decreases tetracycline absorption. There are no clinically significant drug-to-food/herbal interactions established for riopan. Drug-to-drug interactions may occur with the simultaneous use of phenytoin or chloramphenicol with *folic acid*, both of which may increase the metabolism of folic acid and decrease its levels. There are no clinically significant drug-to-herbal interactions established.

With *hydrochlorothiazide*, drug-to-drug interactions may occur with the simultaneous use of other potassium-wasting diuretics, which may increase hypokalemic effects. When used with corticosteroids there is an increased risk of hyperglycemia. Cholestyramine and colestipol decrease thiazide absorption. Allopurinol may increase the risk of hypersensitivity reactions. Drug-to-food/herbal interactions may occur with the simultaneous use of licorice and stimulant laxative herbs (aloe, cascara, sagada, senna), which may increase the risk of potassium depletion. Simultaneous use with gingko may decrease antihypertensive effects. Drug-to-drug interactions may occur with the simultaneous use of *phytonadione* antibiotics, warfarin, cholestyramine, colestipol, sucralfate, and mineral oil, all of which may decrease absorption of oral phytondione. Quinidine, high-dose salicylates, and sulfonamides increase the requirements for vitamin K. There are no clinically significant drug-to-food/herbal interactions established. Drug-to-drug interactions may occur with the simultaneous use of *diphenhydramine HcL* and central nervous system (CNS) depressants, alcohol, antianxiolytics, antidepressants, other antihistamines, opioid analgesics, and sedative/hypnotics, which may increase CNS depression. Simultaneous use with MAO inhibitors increases the risk of hypertensive crisis. Drug-to-herbal interactions may occur with the simultaneous use of kava, valerian, skullcap, chamomile, or hops, which can increase CNS depression.

9. Discuss alternative invasive procedures that may be implemented if drug therapy fails to control the presenting symptoms of cirrhosis of the liver.

- Abdominal paracentesis is the aspiration of fluid from the peritoneal cavity to relieve severe ascites that does not respond to diuretic therapy. The client signs an informed consent and is weighed, and vital signs are taken. The client voids immediately prior to the procedure to avoid bladder puncture. The client then sits in a chair or on the side of the bed in an upright position with feet supported. The upright position allows the intestines to float back and away from the insertion site, thus avoiding puncture. Blood pressure is monitored during the procedure. The area of insertion is cleansed with antibacterial agent (e.g., betadine), local anesthesia is administered at the site, an incision is made, and a needle or a trocar is inserted to withdraw fluid to send to the laboratory to be analyzed. After the needle is withdrawn, a small dressing is placed over the puncture site. Salt-poor albumin may be administered after the procedure to replace lost proteins.
- Peritoneovenous shunt is a surgical procedure that provides continuous reinfusion of ascitic fluid into the venous system. One type, the LaVeen peritoneovenous shunt, consists of a tube and a one-way valve. The tube runs from the abdominal cavity through the peritoneum, under the subcutaneous tissue, and into the jugular vein or superior

vena cava. The valve opens when the pressure in the peritoneal cavity is three to five cm H_2O higher than that in the superior vena cava. This allows the ascitic fluid to flow into the venous system. It is the client's inspiration that increases the intraperitoenal pressure, causing the valve to open. The shunting of the fluid causes improvement in hemodynamic factors and increases sodium and fluid excretion, with increase in urinary output.

- Portacaval anastomoses are surgical bypass procedures use to relieve portal hypertension in clients with cirrhosis of the liver. One of these procedures is the portacaval anastomosis, in which portal blood is shunted into the vena cava, resulting in the decrease of pressure in the portal system. When pressure is decreased, the danger of esophageal and gastric varices hemorrhage is reduced. If the portal vein cannot be used, a shunt may be made between the splenic vein and the left renal vein, which is referred to as a splenorenal shunt. A mesocaval shunt is another type of bypass procedure in which the inferior vena cava is severed and the proximal end of the vena cava is anastomosed to the side of the superior mesenteric vein. This type of shunt also lowers pressure in the portal system.

- Transjugular intrahepatic portal-systemic shunt is a nonsurgical procedure in which a tract (shunt) between the systemic and portal venous systems is created to redirect portal blood flow. A catheter is placed in the jugular vein and then threaded through the superior and inferior vena cava to the hepatic vein. The wall of the hepatic vein is punctured, and the catheter is directed to the portal vein. Stents are positioned along the passageway, overlapping in the liver tissue and extending into both veins.

10. If Mr. S develops massive hemorrhage and replacement blood products are not readily available, what alternatives would the health care provider prescribe? The health care provider would prescribe IV fluids, such as 0.9% sodium chloride or fresh frozen plasma. The normal saline expands the intravascular volume and replaces extracellular fluid loss and, in doing so, prevents vascular collapse or hypovolemic shock. The fresh frozen plasma aids in the restoration of clotting factors.

11. If Mr. S develops portal systemic encephalopathy (PSE), what would be the probable treatment plan? Clients with PSE have a high ammonia level because the liver cannot convert the ammonia to a less-toxic form, therefore, ammonia and other by-products of metabolism are carried by the circulatory system to the brain, where they interfere with normal cerebral function. Because ammonia is formed in the gastrointestinal (GI) tract by the action of bacterial on protein, nonsurgical treatments are used to reduce bacterial breakdown. For instance, diet therapy that has simple carbohydrate and

low-protein foods. Drugs to eliminate or reduce ammonia levels include lactulose, a drug that promotes the excretion of ammonia in the stool. The nurse who administers lactulose should monitor the client for complaints of abdominal bloating and cramping, hypokalemia, and dehydration from the excess stool that occurs from the effect of the lactulose. To diminish protein breakdown in the bowel, and decrease the rate of ammonia production, neomycin sulfate, a broad-spectrum antibiotic, is given. It acts as an intestinal antiseptic to destroy the normal flora in the bowel and, in doing so, decreases the rate of ammonia production in the gastrointestinal (GI) tract.

12. Discuss client education for cirrhosis of the liver. Alcohol abstinence is mandatory. Initiation of detoxification is necessary before discharge from the hospital. The client should consume a diet that adheres to the guidelines set by the health care provider, the nurse, and the dietitian. The client should be instructed to eat small, frequent meals that are nutritionally well balanced. Compliance with medication therapy is vital, so clients should be taught to take all medications as prescribed, and to not take any other medications unless specifically prescribed by the health care provider. Maintaining follow-up care as instructed should be stressed. Clients in need of assistance in dealing with alcohol abstinence can be referred to Alcoholics Anonymous, and the American Liver Foundation is an excellent source for information about liver disease.

References

Broyles, B. E. (2005). *Medical-Surgical Nursing Clinical Companion*. Durham, NC: Carolina Academic Press.

Corbet, J. V. (2004). *Laboratory Tests and Diagnostic Procedures with Nursing Diagnoses* (6th ed.). Upper Saddle River, NJ: Prentice Hall.

Gahart, B. L. and Nazareno, A. R. (2005). *2005 Intravenous Medications*. St. Louis: Mosby.

Heitz, U. and Horne, M. M. (2005). *Mosby's Pocket Guide Series: Fluid, Electrolyte, and Acid-Base Balance* (5th ed.). St. Louis: Mosby.

Huether, S. E. and McCance (2004). *Understanding Pathophysiology* (3rd ed.). St. Louis: Mosby.

Ignatavicius, D. D. and Workman, M. L. (2006). *Medical-Surgical Nursing across the Health Care Continuum* (5th ed.). Philadelphia: W. B. Saunders.

Lewis, S. M., Heitkemper, M. M., and Dirksen, S. R. (2004). *Medical-Surgical Nursing* (6th ed.). Philadelphia: Mosby.

Smeltzer, S. C. and Bare, B. G. (2005). *Medical-Surgical Nursing* (7th ed.). Philadelphia: Lippincott Williams & Wilkins.

Spratto, G. R. and Woods, A. L. (2005). *2005 Edition: PDR Nurse's Drug Handbook*. Clifton Park, NY: Thomson Delmar Learning.

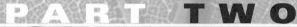

PART TWO

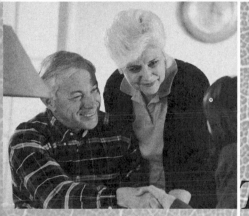

The Respiratory and Immune Systems

Acute Bacterial (Streptococcal) Pneumonia

GENDER

M

AGE

65

SETTING

- Adult home/hospital

ETHNICITY/CULTURE

- White American

PREEXISTING CONDITIONS

COEXISTING CONDITIONS

- Recent respiratory infection

LIFESTYLE

- Retired bus operator for private company

COMMUNICATION

DISABILITY

- Inability to do activities of daily living (ADLs)

SOCIOECONOMIC STATUS

- Low

SPIRITUAL/RELIGIOUS

- Lutheran

PHARMACOLOGIC

- Cefuroxime sodium (Zinacef)
- Acetaminophen (Tylenol, suppository)

PSYCHOSOCIAL

- Anxiety

LEGAL

ETHICAL

- Room at adult home may not be available upon discharge

ALTERNATIVE THERAPY

PRIORITIZATION

- Antibiotic therapy

DELEGATION

- RN
- Client education

THE RESPIRATORY AND IMMUNE SYSTEMS

Level of difficulty: Easy

Overview: This case involves critical assessment to identify the severity of symptoms and the need for competence in maintaining thermo-regulation, relieving pleuritic chest pain, and stabilizing effective airway maintenance. The case also involves prioritization in triage situations in a busy emergency department.

Client Profile

Mr. M is a 65-year-old male, 5'5" and 204 pounds. He is a widower who has been living in an adult home since the death of his wife. He has no children but speaks of a younger brother with whom he has not communicated for the past ten years.

Case Study

Mr. M is seen in the emergency department (ED) with sudden onset of shaking chills, a fever of 103.6° F, complaints of stabbing chest pain that is aggravated by increased respirations, and coughing. He reports years of cigarette smoking, of which he reports decreasing from four packs to one pack per day. In discussing his social habits, he reports enjoying being alone in his room, watching television or listening to radio programs. He admits to having a good appetite but prefers to eat late at night, to which he attributes the excess weight. He says his meals consist mostly of fast food, because this adult home does not provide meals. He denies any present medications, including herbal or over-the-counter (OTC) medications, and has not had any vaccines for several years. Mr. M is triaged and transferred to the medical intensive care unit (MICU). On arrival to the MICU, he manifested marked tachypnea (25 to 45/min), accompanied by respiratory grunting, nasal flaring, and the use of accessory muscles of respiration and pulse rate of 110 and bounding. He requests being propped up in bed but occasionally leans forward as he tries to cough and breathe deeply. He is perspiring profusely. The resident health care provider visits with Mr. M and prescribes 2 liters of oxygen via nasal cannula, which was initiated. The history and physical was delayed until Mr. M was more stabilized. He is to remain on bed rest with oxygen in progress. His current vital signs:

Blood pressure: 124/78
Pulse: 98
Respirations: 30
Temperature: 102° F

Sputum and blood for culture and sputum for gram stain, chest X-ray and pulmonary function tests, complete blood count (CBC), and blood urea nitrogen (BUN) are ordered and done. Pulse oximeter reading is 89%. Acetaminophen suppository is administered, and the client is placed on a cooling blanket, as prescribed by the nurse practitioner (NP) of the unit. A health care provider sees Mr. M at a later time, the history and physical examination are done and lab results reviewed. The blood culture and sputum specimen is positive for Staphylococcus aureus. The chest X-ray shows consolidation of the lungs. Pulmonary function tests reveal decreased lung volumes and decreased compliance with increased airway resistance. The CBC reveals:

> White blood cell (WBC) count: $12,000/mm^3$
> Blood urea nitrogen (BUN): 30 mg/dL

After the interdisciplinary team reviews the diagnostic studies and signs and symptoms of the client on admission, a diagnosis of acute bacterial pneumonia is confirmed.

Questions

1. Discuss different classification of pneumonia.

2. Discuss the most common community-acquired pneumonia for clients younger than 60 years of age without comorbidity and those older than 60 years of age with comorbidity, and why this trend occurs.

3. Discuss the pathogenesis of pneumococcal pneumonia.

4. Identify the common organisms responsible for hospital-acquired pneumonia (HAP).

5. Discuss methicillin-resistant S. aureus.

6. What are the purposes for the prescribed orders?

7. What are the most common adverse reactions, drug-to-drug, drug-to-food/herbal interactions of the prescribed medications?

8. Discuss nursing diagnoses, outcomes, and interventions for pneumonia.

9. Discuss the gerontological considerations for elderly clients with pneumonia.

10. Discuss promotion of home- and community-based care for the client with pneumonia.

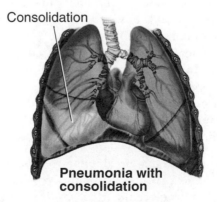

Consolidation

**Pneumonia with
consolidation**

Pneumonia with consolidation will create a crackling sound or occasional friction rub.

Questions and Suggested Answers

1. **Discuss different classification of pneumonia.** Classification of pneumonia is important because of differences in the likely causative organisms

and the selection of appropriate antibiotics. Classification of pneumonia includes community acquired pneumonia (CAP), which is due to a lower respiratory tract infection of the lung with onset in the community during the first two days of hospitalization. The incidence in the United States is increasing; 6.5 million adults develop CAP annually, 1.5 million of whom are eventually hospitalized. Its incidence is highest in the winter months, and smoking is an important risk factor. An organism commonly identified in CAP is Staphylococcus (S.) pneumoniae.

Hospital-acquired pneumonia (HAP) is pneumonia that occurs 48 hours or longer after hospital admission. It is estimated to occur at a rate of 5 to 10 cases per 1,000 hospital admissions. Bacteria that are responsible for HAP infections include pseudomonas, enterobacter, S. aureus, and S. pneumoniae. Many of the organisms causing HAP enter the lungs after aspiration of particles from the client's own pharynx.

Aspiration pneumonia refers to the sequelae occurring from abnormal entry of secretions or substances into the lower airway. It usually follows aspiration of material from the mouth or stomach into the trachea and, subsequently, the lungs. The person who has aspiration pneumonia usually has a history of lost consciousness (e.g., as a result of seizure, anesthesia, head injury, stroke, and alcohol intake). Because these persons usually have depressed gag reflex, aspiration is more likely to occur. Another risk factor for aspiration pneumonia is tube feedings, with the dependent portions of the lung most often affected.

Opportunistic pneumonia is used in reference to persons who are highly susceptible to respiratory infections, those who have severe protein-calorie malnutrition, those who have immune deficiencies, those who have received transplants, and those who have been treated with immunosuppressive drugs. Another group includes persons who are treated with radiation therapy, chemotherapy drugs, and corticosteroids for prolonged periods of time. An example of an opportunistic pneumonia is pneumocystitis carinii, an opportunistic pathogen whose natural habitat is the lung. It affects 70% of persons with human immunodeficiency virus (HIV) and is the most common opportunistic infection in clients with acquired immunodeficiency syndrome (AIDS).

2. Discuss the most common community-acquired pneumonia for clients younger than 60 years of age without comorbidity and those older than 60 years of age with comorbidity, and why this trend occurs? The most common community-acquired pneumonia for these two groups of clients is pneumococcal pneumonia, also called bacterial pneumonia. Its presentation is usually acute, with rapid onset of shaking chills, fever, and cough productive of rust-colored or purulent sputum. It usually resolves uneventfully, with normal lung structure restored upon completion of the process. Its most common completion is infection involving the pleurae (pleuritis).

3. Discuss the pathogenesis of pneumococcal pneumonia. The pathogenesis of pneumococcal pneumonia begins with the aspiration of S. pneumonia into the lungs; an inflammatory response is initiated resulting in alveolar edema and exudate formation. As the disease progresses, alveoli and respiratory bronchioles fill with serous exudate, blood cells, fibrin, and bacteria. Eventually there is consolidation of lung tissue, which, if it involves an entire lung, is referred to as lobar pneumonia.

4. Identify the common organisms responsible for hospital-acquired pneumonia (HAP). The common organisms are enterobacter species, Escherichia coli, Klebsiella species, Proteus, Serratia marcescens, P. aeruginosa, methicillin-sensitive, and methicillin-resistant Staphylococcus aureus (MRSA).

5. Discuss methicillin-resistant Staphylococcus aureus. Methicillin-resistant Staphylococcus aureus (MRSA) is a highly virulent organism, requiring special management techniques. More than 50% of all hospital-acquired S. aureus infections are methicillin resistant. These bacteria are highly adaptable organisms that have acquired resistance through clever mechanisms to evade pharmacologic innovations. Inappropriate antibiotic use has been one of the major factors contributing to the development of drug-resistant organisms. MRSA is spread primarily by direct contact with the hands of health care workers and can remain viable for days on environmental surfaces and clothing.

Nursing management includes teaching staff, client, and significant others that hand-washing remains the first line of defense in preventing the spread of the infection. An antiseptic soap should be used at all times to wash hands so as to kill these bacteria. Contact isolation should be maintained, therefore, the client is placed in a private room and health care providers and significant others should wear gloves at all times when in contact with the immediate environment of the client. If soiling is likely, the care provider should wear a gown. A legible sign indicating that contact isolation is in progress should be placed at the entrance of the client's room. The number of people in contact with clients should be minimized, and appropriate precautions must be taken when transporting clients within or between facilities.

The following are prescribed:

- Cefuroxime sodium (Zinacef) IV 1.5 g q6h
- Tylenol (acetaminophen) suppository for temp greater than 101 stat and q4h PRN
- IV Dextrose 5% and 0.45% sodium chloride at 125 mL/hr

6. What are the purposes for the prescribed orders? *Cefuroxime sodium* is a cephalosporin antibiotic that destroys the S. aureus organism found in the blood culture and sputum specimen. It works by being active against gram-negative and gram-positive aerobic and anaerobic organisms. It inhibits the third and final stage of bacterial cell-wall synthesis, thus promoting loss of membrane integrity, which leads to death of the organism. *Acetaminophen suppository* is an antipyretic and non-opioid analgesic that lowers the temperature. Acetaminophen lowers fever by direct action on hypothalmus heat-regulating center with consequent peripheral vasodilation, sweating, and dissipation of heat. *D5%W/45% NS* at 125 mL/hr rehydrate the client by replenishing insensible loss due to diaphoresis related to the elevated temperature. The glucose in the intravenous fluid provides energy that is needed, because pneumonia process depletes the body of energy.

7. **What are the most common adverse reactions, drug-to-drug, drug-to-food/herbal interactions of the prescribed medications?** The most common adverse reactions of *cefuroxime sodium* are hypersensitivity responses, rashes, abdominal pain, diarrhea, nausea, gastrointestinal tract irritation, and phlebitis at the peripheral site of the infusion, especially if the drug is infused too rapidly for the access.

Drug-to-drug interactions may occur with the simultaneous use of probenecid, which decreases excretion and increases blood levels of renal excreted cephalosporins. Concurrent use with aminoglycosides and loop diuretics may increase the risk of renal toxicity. Cefuroxime may antagonize the effects of chloramphenicol, erythromycin, and tetracyclines. Large doses of cephalosporins and/or salicylates may cause hypoprothrombinemia. Use of nonsteroidal anti-inflammatory agents (NSAIDs), naproxen, or sulfinpyrazone may cause increased risk of bleeding due to their gastrointestinal ulcerative potential.

There are no clinically significant drug-to-food/herbal interactions established. The most common adverse reaction of *acetaminophen* is hepatotoxicity. Drug-to-drug interactions may occur with the simultaneous use of alcohol, sulfinpyrazone, isoniazid, rifampin, rifabutin, phenytoin, barbiturates, and carbamazepine and may increase the risk of acetaminophen-induced liver damage, and increase the therapeutic effects of acetaminophen. Concurrent use with salicylates or NSAIDs increases the risk of adverse renal effects. Concurrent use with propranolol decreases the metabolism of *acetaminophen* and may increase the effects. Concurrent use with lamotrigene, zidovudine, and loop diuretics may decrease their effects. There are no clinically significant drug-to-food interactions, however, use with milk thistle may help prevent acetaminophen liver damage.

8. **Discuss nursing diagnoses, outcomes, and interventions for pneumonia.** *Nursing diagnosis:* Ineffective airway clearance R/T excessive secretions and weak cough.

Expected outcome: The client will maintain effective airway clearance by having a patent airway and effectively clearing secretions.

Nursing intervention: Increase fluid intake if not contraindicated. Teach and encourage effective coughing and deep-breathing techniques, and turn and position the client frequently to aid in the mobilization of secretions. If the client has an altered level of consciousness, turn at least every two hours and place in a side-lying position to prevent aspiration. Administer bronchodilators as prescribed, and perform chest physiotherapy and suctioning as needed.

Nursing diagnosis: Ineffective-breathing pattern R/T tachypnea.

Expected outcome: The client will have improved breathing patterns, as seen with a respiratory rate of 12, adequate chest expansion, clear breath sounds, and decreased dyspnea.

Nursing intervention: Position the client for comfort and to facilitate breathing (e.g., raise the head of the bed 45 degrees). Teach the client how to splint the chest wall with a small pillow to promote comfort during coughing. Administer cough medicine as prescribed, and routinely monitor respiratory rate, auscultate the chest, observe for signs of hypoxemia, utilize the pulse oximeter, and document care provided.

Nursing diagnosis: Activity intolerance R/T decreased oxygen levels for metabolic demands.

Expected outcome: The client will have improved activity tolerance as evidenced by an ability to perform activities of daily living and a progressive increase in physical activities without excessive dyspnea and fatigue.

Nursing intervention: Assess the client's baseline activity level and response to activity, and focus on how well the client tolerates activities. Assess for changes in respiratory and pulse rate, marked dyspnea, fatigue, pallor or cyanosis, and dysrhythmias to determine client's tolerance to activities. Schedule activities after treatments or medications. Balance activity with adequate rest periods.

9. **Discuss the gerontological considerations for elderly clients with pneumonia.** Pneumonia in elderly clients may occur as a primary problem or as a complication of a chronic disease process. Pulmonary infections in the elderly frequently are difficult to treat and have a higher mortality rate than in younger clients. In the older clients, manifestations of pneumonia may be seen with general deterioration, weakness, abdominal symptoms, anorexia, confusion, tachycardia, and tachypnea. The diagnosis of pneumonia in the older clients may be more difficult to diagnose because their immune systems are low, which may mask the classic symptoms of cough, chest pain, sputum production, and fever.

10. Discuss promotion of home- and community-based care for the client with pneumonia. Teach clients the importance of compliance with medication regimen and the importance of completing prescribed medications even when there are no signs or symptoms of the disease process. Teach the adverse effects of prescribed medications (write the effects down as appropriate for the client). Teach the importance of avoiding conditions that increase oxygen demand, such as smoking, temperature extremes, weight gain, and stress. Reinforce the importance of pursed-lip and diaphragmatic breathing, and request return demonstration before client leaves the health care setting. Emphasize the importance of follow-up care with primary health care provider. Emphasize that smoking cessation is mandatory.

References

Broyles, B. E. (2005). *Medical-Surgical Nursing Clinical Companion*. Durham, NC: Carolina Academic Press.

Corbet, J. V. (2004). *Laboratory Tests and Diagnostic Procedures with Nursing Diagnoses*. (6th ed.). Upper Saddle River, NJ: Prentice Hall.

Gahart, B. L. and Nazareno, A. R. (2005). *2005 Intravenous Medications*. St. Louis: Elsevier Mosby.

Heuther, S. E. and McCance, K. L. (2004). *Understanding Pathophysiology* (3rd ed.). St. Louis: Mosby.

Ignatavicius, D. D. and Workman, M. L. (2006). *Medical-Surgical Nursing across the Health Care Continuum* (5th ed.). Philadelphia: W. B. Saunders.

Langford, R. W. and Thompson, J. D. (2005). *Mosby's Handbook of Diseases*. (3rd ed.). St. Louis: Mosby.

Spratto, G. R. and Woods, A. L. (2005). *2005 Edition: PDR Nurse's Drug Handbook*. Clifton Park, NY: Thomson Delmar Learning.

CASE STUDY 2

Acute Asthma

GENDER

F

AGE

30

SETTING

- Hospital asthma clinic

ETHNICITY/CULTURE

- Hispanic

PREEXISTING CONDITIONS

COEXISTING CONDITIONS

- Parents and two of her siblings have asthma

LIFESTYLE

- Full-time college student

COMMUNICATION

- Spanish and English

DISABILITY

SOCIOECONOMIC STATUS

- Middle

SPIRITUAL/RELIGIOUS

- Catholic

PHARMACOLOGIC

- Albuterol (Proventil)
- Metaproterenol sulfate (Alupent)
- Ipratropium bromide (Atrovent)
- Epinephrine (Adrenalin)
- Hydrocortisone (Solu-Cortef)
- Aminophylline (Theophylline ethylenediamine)

PSYCHOSOCIAL

- Anxiety

LEGAL

ETHICAL

ALTERNATIVE THERAPY

PRIORITIZATION

- Maintain airway patency
- Relieve symptoms

DELEGATION

- RN
- CNA
- Client education

MODERATE

THE RESPIRATORY AND IMMUNE SYSTEMS

Level of difficulty: Moderate

Overview: This case involves the use of critical thinking skills and the nursing process to effectively prioritize and delegate care, to maintain optimum airway management, and alleviate symptoms and complications. The registered nurse (RN) can delegate the monitoring of vital signs to the certified nursing attendant.

Client Profile

Ms. A is a 30-year-old female who is accompanied to the outpatient clinic of the hospital by a classmate. On arrival, Ms. A complains of pain in her sinuses and reports headache for two days. While the nurse is collecting the initial data, Ms. A starts sneezing and tells the nurse, "I am having an asthmatic attack, I can feel it coming on." She is anxious with inspiratory-expiratory ratio prolonged at 1:4. Ms. A leans forward as though to enhance her ventilation and is using her accessory muscles of the neck to help with breathing. Ms. A reports allergy to "strong perfumes."

Case Study

Ms. A's vital signs are:

Blood pressure: 150/98
Pulse: 120
Respirations: 22 and shallow
Temperature: 98.4° F

Ms. A is initially seen in the triage area of the emergency department (ED) by a nurse practitioner (NP), who notifies the ED health care provider of Ms. A's arrival and presenting symptoms. The health care provider responds and arrives in the triage area within minutes.

Ms. A is in the early-phase of asthmatic attack, with complaints of spasms in the chest, complaints of chest tightness, and audible wheezing. Ms. A is dyspneic and is coughing even though she is in a high-Fowler's position. Metaproterenol (Alupent) nebulizer five inhalations of undiluted 5% solution and an intravenous line is initiated with D5%W at 100 mL/hr. An arterial blood gas (ABG) is done and reveals a pH 7.48, pO_2 of 90, PCO_2 and HCO_3 22, and sputum and blood tests reveal elevated levels of eosinophils and elevated IgE. Oxygen two liters via nasal cannula is initiated. Ms. A continues to complain of chest tightness. A stat dose of ipratropium bromide (Atrovent) is administered, and aminophylline IV will be initiated as per the health care provider's verbal suggestion.

The triage nurse assigns a licensed practical nurse (LPN) to remain with the client, while the registered nurse attends to other, critically ill clients. The health care provider arrives just when the client begins to progress to status asthmaticus. Epinephrine 0.5 mL of 1:1000 SC is administered by the health care provider, which results in temporary relief of the symptoms. An order is also written for hydrocortisone 100 mg IV bolus in 50 mL D5%W stat.

The health care provider completes the physical assessment, and Ms. A is transferred to a respiratory care unit of the hospital. Ms. A is placed in high-Fowler's, oxygen is increased to four liters via NC as prescribed, and intravenous fluids of D5%W at 100 mL/hr are initiated. On arrival to the respiratory unit, ABG and serum labs are drawn and sent to the lab stat. The lab results are:

Glucose: 108 mg/dL
Blood urea nitrogen (BUN): 15 mg/dL
Creatinine: 0.7 mg/dL
Sodium (Na): 138 mEq/L
Potassium (K+): 4.3 mEq/L
White blood cell (WBC) count: 7.4 mm/^{3}
Red blood cell (RBC) count: 4.21
Hemoglobin (Hgb): 13.5 g/dL
Hematocrit (Hct): 34.8%
Platelet count: 273,000/mm^3
Initial pulse oximeter reading: 97%
Current arterial blood gas (ABG): pH 7.48, pO$_2$ 98 mm Hg, pCO$_2$ 60 mm Hg and HCO$_3$ 22 mEq
Pulmonary function tests: PEFR 94 ml/L
Forced expiratory volume/forced vital capacity (FEV$_1$/FVC): 68

Albuterol nebulizer is administered and repeat FEV$_1$/FVC shows an increase of 78%. ABG will be implemented as needed. After the health care provider reviewed the diagnostic report and subjective and objective data, a diagnosis of asthma is confirmed.

Questions

1. What is your understanding of the above situation?

2. Discuss the cells that play a key role in the inflammation of asthma?

3. Identify and discuss the three most common symptoms of asthma.

4. What are the comorbid conditions that may accompany asthma?

5. What are the common nursing diagnoses for clients with acute asthma?

6. What are the purposes for the prescribed orders?

7. What are the most common adverse reactions of the prescribed medications?

8. Discuss the drug-to-drug, drug-to-food/herbal interactions for the prescribed medications?

9. Discuss the key complications of asthma?

10. If Ms. A develops status asthmaticus, what would be the medical management in order of priority?

11. Discuss Peak Flow Monitoring and its benefits in acute asthma.

12. Discuss home and community-based care for clients with history of asthma who need to provide self-care.

Questions and Suggested Answers

1. **What is your understanding of the above situation?** Ms. A may have come in contact with other allergens she is not aware of over the past two days, or the reaction may be due to sinusitis which has manifested itself in the form of pain in her sinuses, and headache. Allergy is the strongest predisposing factor for asthma. Ms. A may have been exposed to an allergen in the outpatient clinic where many clients and families gather. Someone in the outpatient clinic may have used a strong perfume that has caused Ms. A to develop an allergic reaction. Bronchial asthma is an intermittent and reversible airflow obstruction affecting only the airways, not the alveoli. Different types of events are known to trigger asthmatic attacks.

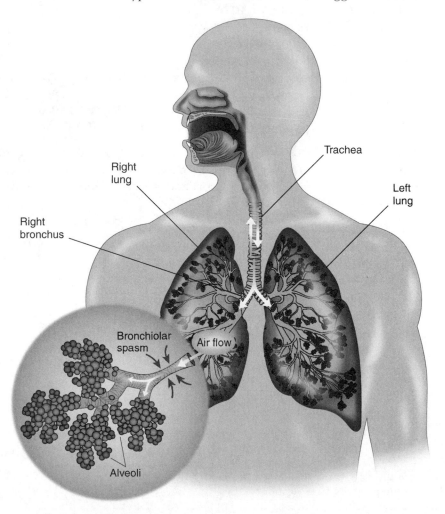

Asthma involves bronchospasm and excessive airway secretions.

Inflammation of the mucous membrane lining the airways is a key event in triggering the presence of specific allergens; nonallergenic general irritants such as cold air, dry air, or fine airborne particles, odors, microorganisms, and aspirin are known to trigger bronchial asthma.

2. **Discuss the cells that play a key role in the inflammation of asthma?** Mast cells are large cells with cytoplasmic granules that contain an abundant mixture of chemical mediators, including histamine, which is a vasoactive amine that acts rapidly to make local blood vessels more permeable such as in asthmatic attacks that occur with an inflammatory response. Histamine causes capillary leak, which results in mast cells continuing to release histamine and other proteins, prolonging the response of the inflammatory process. The continued inflammatory process further obstructs airways by constricting bronchial smooth muscle, causing a narrowing of the airway from the outside, resulting in bronchiolar hyperresponsiveness and clinical manifestations such as bronchospasms, audible wheezing, and increased respiratory rate.

- Neutrophils are the predominant and first phagocytic cells to arrive at the inflamed site to ingest bacteria, dead cells, and cellular debris that may occur with the inflammatory process that occurs with asthma.
- Macrophages are the next phagocytes to arrive at the site of inflammation, and perform the same function as neutrophils. However, macrophages remain for a longer time during the inflammatory process.
- Eosinophils respond to the inflammatory process and help to control the inflammatory response.
- Lymphocytes such as sensitized T and B-lymphocytes form IgE antibodies in response to an allergen-antibody mechanism that occurs with asthmatic attacks. During an asthmatic attack, the allergen-antibody mechanism causes the release of chemical mediators that create the inflammatory response. The IgE antibodies that are formed by the T and B lymphocytes circulate and attach themselves to mast cells, resulting in the release of different chemical mediators such as histamine, which cause temporary and rapid constriction of smooth muscles, with production of excess mucus.

3. **Identify and discuss the three most common symptoms of asthma.** The three most common symptoms of asthma are cough, dyspnea, and wheezing. In some instances, cough may be the only symptom, and may be with or without mucus production. At times the mucus is so tightly wedged in the narrow airway that the client cannot cough it up. Wheezing may be generalized, first on expiration and then possibly during inspiration as well, and generalized chest tightness and dyspnea occur.

4. What are the comorbid conditions that may accompany asthma? Gastroesophageal reflux (GER) is any clinically significant symptomatic condition or histopathologic alteration presumed to be secondary to reflux of gastric contents into the lower esophagus. Its relationship with asthma is not researched proven at this time. However, it is believed that reflux of stomach acid into the esophagus can be aspirated into the lungs, causing reflex vagal stimulation and bronchoconstriction. It is also believed that GER is primarily involved in nocturnal asthma, but it can trigger daytime asthma as well. The monitoring of esophageal pH simultaneously with peak expiratory flow rate (PEFR) can determine if this is the cause of asthma.

- Drug-induced asthma may occur from certain drugs such as aspirin, nonsteroidal inflammatory drugs (e.g., ibuprofen [Motrin], indomethacin [Indocin]), B-adrenergic blockers (e.g., propranolol [Inderal], timolol [Timoptic]), which may trigger asthma because they inhibit adrenergic stimulation of the bronchioles and in doing so prevent bronchodilation.
- Allergic bronchopulmonary aspergillosis. Aspergillosis is a fungus that if inhaled can cause inflammatory granulomatous lesions in the bronchioles. If this inflammatory process occurs, it may require treatment with corticosteroids instead of the usual bronchodilating drugs used to treat asthmatic occurrences.

5. What are the common nursing diagnoses for clients with acute asthma?
- Ineffective airway clearance R/T bronchospasms, ineffective cough, excessive mucus production, tenacious secretions, and fatigue
- Anxiety R/T difficulty breathing, perceived or actual loss of control, and fear of suffocation
- Ineffective therapeutic regimen management R/T lack of information about asthma and its treatment

The following are prescribed:

- Albuterol (Proventil) two puffs stat
- Metaproterenol sulfate (Alupent) nebulization: three inhalations q3h
- Ipratropium bromide (Atrovent) three puffs q6h for bronchospasms
- Epinephrine (Adrenalin) 0.5 mL of 1:1000 SC stat
- Hydrocortisone (Solu-Cortef) 100 mg IV in 50 mL of D5%W stat
- Aminophylline (Theophylline ethylenediamine) 1 g in 100 mL D5%W, infuse for one hour

6. What are the purposes for the prescribed orders? *Metaproterenol* is a direct-acting sympathominetic that stimulates the beta-2 receptors causing relaxation of the smooth muscle of the bronchi resulting in bronchodilation. *Ipratropium bromide* is a cholinergic blocking agent chemically related to atropine sulfate. It prevents increased levels of cyclic guanosine

monophosphate that cause bronchoconstriction. *Aminophylline* is a respiratory stimulant and potent bronchodilator used to treat the bronchoconstriction characteristic of asthma exacerbation. *Epinephrine* is a sympathomimetic agent that causes marked stimulation of the alpha, beta-1, and beta-2 receptors resulting in bronchodilation and decongestion. It is a first line agent for severe asthma exacerbation. *Hydrocortisone* is an adrenoglucocorticoid anti-inflammatory that is administered to decrease the inflammatory response that occurs in asthma exacerbation or status asthmaticus. Intravenous infusion of hydrocortisone results in immediate effects because it has the abilities of decreasing synthesis and release of inflammatory mediators such as leukotrienes, histamine and prostaglandins; decreasing infiltration and activity of inflammatory cells such as eosinophils, and leukocytes; and decreasing edema of the airway mucosa. By suppressing inflammation, hydrocortisone reduces bronchial hyperreactivity, and enhances airway effectiveness. *Albuterol* nebulizers are used for their sympathomimetic effects causing bronchodilation.

7. **What are the most common adverse reactions of the prescribed medications?** The most common adverse effect of *metaproterenol sulfate* is tachycardia. By stimulating the beta-2 receptors that also are present in the heart, it causes the heart rate to increase. The most common adverse effects of *ipratropium bromide* are tachycardia, nervousness, dizziness, headache, difficulty in coordination, and drowsiness. The most common adverse effects of intravenous *aminophylline* include tachycardia, headache, insomnia, nausea, and vomiting occurring when peak serum concentrations are less than 20 mcg/mL. Toxicity can occur with concentrations greater than 20 mcg/ml and can result in severe bronchoconstriction. Due to the stimulant effects of *epinephrine* the most common adverse effect is tachycardia. Others include hypertension, anxiety, and the potential for life-threatening ventricular fibrillation, cerebral or subarachnoid hemorrhage, and angina pectoris. Adverse effects of *parenteral hydrocortisone* are rare with only one injection. Long-term use can result in altered glucose metabolism, increasing serum glucose levels, Cushing's syndrome, electrolyte and calcium imbalance, increased intraocular pressure, and increased risk of infection. The most common adverse effects of *albuterol* nebulizer doses are tachycardia, nervousness, palpitations, and anxiety.

8. **Discuss the drug-to-drug, drug-to-food/herbal interactions of the prescribed medications?** Drug-to-drug interactions can occur if *metaproterenol sulfate* is administered before or after other sympathomimetic bronchodilators potentiating their action. There are no clinically significant drug-to-food/herbal interactions. With *ipratropium bromide* drug-to-drug interactions can occur with the simultaneous use of amantadine, tricyclic antidepressants, antihistamines benzodiazepines, disopyramide, MAO inhibitors,

meperidine, methylphenidate, nitrates, nitrites, phenothiazines, primidone, procainamide, quinidine, other sympathomimetics, and thoxanthines by increasing the anticholinergic effects. Antacids decrease the absorption of ipratropium from the gastrointestinal system, and increase the drug effects of digoxin and cyclopropane. The use of corticosteroid results in additive increased intraocular pressure when used with ipratropium. If used with haloperidol there is a risk of worsening schizophrenic symptoms. Currently there are no clinically significant drug-to-food/herbal interactions established. With *aminophylline* drug-to-drug interactions can occur with alcohol, allopurinol, and beta-adrenergic blocking agents such as propranolol, cimetidine, clarithromycin, ciprofloxacin, disulfiram, erythromycin, estrogen-containing oral contraceptives, fluvoxamine, interferon alfa-A, methotrexate, mexiletine, pentoxifylline, ticlopidine, troleandomycin, and verapamil, because these agents increase the clearance and consequently decrease the serum levels of aminophylline. Aminophylline can decrease the effects of benzodiazepines and lithium. Carbamazepine and loop diuretics may increase or decrease serum aminophylline levels. There are no clinically significant drug-to-food/herbal interactions established. With **epinephrine** drug-to-drug interactions may occur with the simultaneous use of antihistamines and levothyroxine that increase epinephrine effects. Alpha-adrenergic blocking agents. Ergot alkaloids, nitrites, and phenothiazines can cause a reversal of epinephrine's effects. No clinically significant drug-to-food/herbal interactions have been established. With *hydrocortisone* drug-to-drug interactions can occur with simultaneous use of alcohol, barbiturates, hydantoins, and rifampin that increase metabolism and decrease the effects of hydrocortisone. The risk of hypokalemia increases with the concurrent use of amphotericin B and potassium-depleting diuretics, which also increases the risk of digoxin toxicity. Hydrocortisone may decrease the effectiveness of potassium supplements and antagonize the effects of anticholinesterases, isoniazid, salicylates, and somatrem. It may increase the effects of estrogen-containing oral contraceptives and ketoconazole. For clients receiving insulin, dose adjustments may be required. No clinically significant drug-to-food/herbal interactions have been established. Drug-to-drug/food/herbal interactions occurring with *albuterol* are the same as those for ipratropium bromide. Frequently albuterol and ipratropium bromide are administered in a combined form to increase the bronchodilating effects of these agents.

9. Discuss the key complications of asthma?

- Status asthmaticus is a severe, life-threatening asthma attack that is refractory to usual treatment and places the client at risk for developing respiratory failure. Status asthmaticus manifests itself with bronchospasm and acute airway inflammation, with mucus plugging, edema, and cellular infiltration leading to further airway narrowing.

If there is partial obstruction creates a "ball-valve" effect leading to segmental hyperinflation, which may become extreme and compromise effective tidal volume (the amount of air inhaled and exhaled during normal ventilation).

- Respiratory failure is a condition that occurs as a result of one or more diseases involving the lungs or other body systems. Respiratory failure as a complication may develop due to untreated bronchospasm that interferes with gas exchange, thereby compromising lung ventilation. Clients with asthma are at risk for hypercapnic respiratory failure because the underlying pathophysiology of asthma results in airflow obstruction and air trapping. Hypercapnic respiratory failure results from an imbalance between ventilatory supply, which is the maximum ventilation that a client can sustain without developing respiratory muscle fatigue, and ventilatory demand which is the amount of ventilation needed to keep the $PaCO_2$ within normal limits.
- Aspiration pneumonia may develop due to strenuous coughing and the compromised airway, resulting in secretions entering the lungs. If the aspirated materials contain toxic fluids such as gastric juices, there is chemical injury to the lung. If the organism is one of the normal oropharyngeal flora, sputum for culture and sensitivity is prescribed, and antibiotic therapy is based on the type of organism identified.
- Pneumothorax refers to air in the pleural space that can result in partial or complete collapse of a lung due to accumulation of air in the pleural space. Treatment of a pneumothorax depends on the stability of the client, and the amount of air in the intrapleural space. If the amount of air is minimal, no treatment may be needed, as the pneumothorax will resolve spontaneously. If there is sufficient air to cause intolerable symptoms, the pleural space can be aspirated with a large-bore needle. A Heimlich valve may also be used to evacuate air from the pleural space.

10. If Ms. A develops status asthmaticus, what would be the medical management in order of priority? If a client arrives to the emergency department (ED) in status asthmaticus, the health care provider (health care provider or nurse practitioner) will immediately prescribe intravenous fluids (e.g., 0.9% sodium chloride), systemic quick acting bronchodilators such as albuterol (Proventil), to dilate the bronchioles and help improve breathing; steroids such as prednisolone (Delta-Cortef), epinephrine (Adrenalin) to activate beta-2 receptors the lung, which will promote bronchodilation and improve ventilation. Oxygen to replenish oxygen stores and decreases oxygen demand to avoid further complication such as respiratory failure.

11. Discuss Peak Flow Monitoring and its benefits for acute asthma. Peak Flow meters measure the highest airflow during a forced expiration, and guide management of asthmatic attack. Volume is measured in color-coded zones, with the different colors indicating the client's level of performance. Daily Peak Flow Monitoring is recommended for all clients with moderate or severe asthma, because it helps measure asthma severity. The client is to be instructed in the proper technique. The client's "personal best" is determined after monitoring peak flows for two or three weeks after receiving optimal asthma therapy. The nurse should explain that the green indicates personal best (80–100%), yellow (60–80%), and red (less than 60%). Understanding of the zones will enable the client to monitor and manipulate his or her own therapy, and will also reinforce compliance and independence.

12. Discuss home and community-based care for clients with history of asthma who need to provide self-care. A major challenge is to implement basic asthma management principles at the community level. However, the key issues that need implementation include education of health care providers, establishment of programs for asthma education, use of outpatient follow-up care for clients, and a focus on chronic management versus acute episodic care. Areas of focus for asthma management include avoiding potential environmental asthma triggers, avoid medications that could trigger asthmatic attack such as aspirin, avoid foods that have been prepared with monosodiumglutamate (MSG). The client should be taught to seek medical emergency care if he or she experiences the following: gray or blue fingertips, difficulty breathing, walking or talking, retractions of the neck, chest, or ribs, nasal flaring, failure of medications to control worsening symptoms, and peak expiratory flow rate declining steadily after treatment or flow rate of 50% or below his or her usual flow rate.

References

Broyles, B. E. (2005). *Medical-Surgical Nursing Clinical Companion*. Durham, NC: Carolina Academic Press.

Corbet, J. V. (2004). *Laboratory Tests and Diagnostic Procedures with Nursing Diagnoses* (6th ed.). Upper Saddle River, NJ: Prentice Hall.

Gahart, B. L. and Nazareno, A. R. (2005). *2005 Intravenous Medications*. St. Louis: Elsevier Mosby.

Ignatavicius, D. D. and Workman, M. L. (2006). *Medical-Surgical Nursing Across the Health Care Continuum* (5th ed.). Philadelphia: W. B. Saunders.

Lewis, S. M., Heitkemper McLean, M., and Dirksen, S. R. (2004). *Medical-Surgical Nursing* (6th ed.). St. Louis: Mosby.

Spratto, G. R. and Woods, A. L. (2005). *2005 Edition: PDR Nurse's Drug Handbook*. Clifton Park, NY: Thomson Delmar Learning.

CASE STUDY 3

Pulmonary Embolism

GENDER
- F

AGE
- 70

SETTING
- Nursing home to hospital

ETHNICITY/CULTURE
- Black American

PREEXISTING CONDITIONS

COEXISTING CONDITIONS
- Prolonged immobilization

LIFESTYLE
- Retired housewife

COMMUNICATION

DISABILITY

SOCIOECONOMIC STATUS
- Low

SPIRITUAL/RELIGIOUS
- Baptist

PHARMACOLOGIC
- Enoxaparin (Lovenox)
- Heparin sodium IV
- Warfarin sodium (Coumadin)

PSYCHOSOCIAL
- Anxiety
- Fear

LEGAL

ETHICAL

ALTERNATIVE THERAPY

PRIORITIZATION
- Pain assessment
- EKG
- Prepare for pulmonary angiogram
- Anticoagulation

DELEGATION
- RN
- LPN
- CNA

MODERATE

THE RESPIRATORY AND IMMUNE SYSTEMS

Level of difficulty: Moderate

Overview: This case involves a thorough assessment of the client's condition, including sudden onset of respiratory difficulty, and questioning the client about past medical and surgical problems and medications she may be taking currently. The nurse must use critical thinking and prioritization in the emergency department (ED) so the most critical clients are transferred to a critical care unit for ongoing direct care. The licensed practical nurse (LPN) can continue with assessment after the registered nurse (RN) has initiated the process. The certified nursing assistant (CNA) can collect vital signs and gather equipment as needed.

Client Profile

Mrs. W is a 70-year-old female who is brought via private ambulance from a nursing home to the ED because of sudden onset chest pain and difficulty breathing. On arrival to the ED, the client reports a pain of 4 on a scale of 0–10. A triage nurse initiates assessment, places the client in an upright position, and implements oxygen therapy as per the ED protocol. The client's vital signs are:

Blood pressure: 104/72
Pulse: 98 and bounding
Respirations: 24
Temperature: 99.8° F

Case Study

The ED health care provider reviews Mrs. W's medical records brought by the ambulance personnel. The records reveal the client had surgery of the left hip six months ago and bacterial pneumonia three months ago. An additional report indicates that Mrs. W is assisted to a wheelchair three times a day and attends recreational and physical therapy sessions three times per week. Prior to summoning the ambulance, Mrs. W was in the dining room awaiting her evening meal. It is at this time that she called out to a nursing attendant, indicating that she was having pain in the chest. Mrs. W was assessed by a licensed practical nurse (LPN) assigned to the dining area, while a nursing attendant paged the nursing supervisor. The supervisor responded to the call and, upon arriving to the dining room, found Mrs. W restless, apprehensive, and consistently coughing.

A private ambulance was called (protocol of the nursing home), and the client was taken to the hospital accompanied by an LPN. On arrival to the ED, the client is taken to the triage area, and an immediate transfer of information is done between the triage nurse, the ambulance personnel, and the LPN. The triage nurse identifies the urgency in caring for the client and directs the ED unit clerk to inform the intensive care unit (ICU) that the client will be transferred to the ICU after the ED health care provider evaluates her. The triage nurse continues with the physical assessment and finds tachypnea, crackles over the lung field, S_3 and S_4 heart sounds. A stat arterial blood gas (ABG) is done and reveals respiratory alkalosis, pH 7.48, HCO_3 20 mEq/L, PaO_2 78, $PaCO_2$ 38. Pulse oximeter reveals hypoxemia, and a stat chest X-ray shows bilateral infiltrate is normal. Lasix 40 mg IV is given and chest X-ray is to be repeated later today.

Mrs. W is transferred to the medical intensive care unit (MICU). During the exchange of reports between the ED nurse and the MICU nurse, Mrs. W complains of chest pain that is more painful when she inhales. She is transferred to a bed as the nurse monitors her breathing pattern and repositions her in high-Fowler's. Mrs. W reports that the reposition relieves the pain. Oxygen is maintained at four liters via nasal cannula, and the client remains on bed rest as per the protocol. The nurse practitioner orders a ventilation-perfusion scan (V/Q lung scan). The V/Q scan reveals decreased blood flow in areas of the lung. After a multidisciplinary team reviews subjective and objective data, lab values, and report of the V/Q scan, a diagnosis of pulmonary embolism (PE) is confirmed, with plans to order a spiral computed tomography (CT) depending on Mrs. W's response to the planned medical regimen. A repeat chest X-ray shows a decrease in bilateral infitrates of the lungs. Repeat chest X-rays and diuretics will be administered as needed, and complete blood count, serum sodium, and potassium levels will be ordered.

Questions

1. Discuss your understanding of the above situation.

2. Discuss the incidence and etiological responses for pulmonary embolism (PE).

3. Discuss the most common clinical manifestations of PE.

4. Discuss the complications of PE.

5. Discuss diagnostic studies or serum lab used to confirm PE.

6. What are common nursing diagnoses for clients with PE?

7. What are the purposes for the prescribed orders?

8. What are the most common adverse reactions, drug-to-drug, drug-to-food/herbal interactions for the prescribed medications?

9. Discuss three surgical procedures a health care provider may anticipate for a client with multiple large pulmonary emboli if fibrinolytic therapy is contraindicated.

10. Discuss client education for someone being discharged following successful treatment for a PE.

Questions and Suggested Answers

1. **Discuss your understanding of the above situation.** Mrs. W is a 70-year-old client who is regarded as someone who is advanced in age, which is one of the risk factors for PE. As a person ages and is less mobile, stasis of blood in the legs and sacral area increases hydrostatic pressure on vein walls, and stasis of venous blood and viscosity of the blood predisposes the client to thrombus formation. Deep vein thrombosis (DVT) can develop when slowed blood flow allows platelets and increased levels of calcium from the bones to come in contact with the intima that lines the vessel. A person

advanced in age and residing in a nursing home may be dependent on assistance for mobilization, and also for increase in fluids as necessary. Both factors predispose the individual to thrombus formation in the lower extremities. A major risk factor for PE is DVT, which occurs when a piece of thrombus breaks free and is carried by veins to the right heart and pulmonary circulation, then lodges in a pulmonary blood vessel, resulting in sudden, sharp pleuritic chest pain, dyspnea, and cough. The auscultating of S_3 and S_4 heart sounds are indications of pending heart failure or the sudden distention of the ventricular walls by blood from the atria. The bilateral infiltrates seen on the chest X-ray may be due to accumulation of fluid due to damage to the pulmonary blood capillary membranes, due to the embolus.

2. Discuss the incidence and etiological responses for pulmonary embolism (PE). PE affects at least 500,000 people per year in the United States, about 10% of whom die. Another 650,000 have nonfatal PEs. Massive emboli may produce sudden collapse of the client with shock, pallor, severe dyspnea, and crushing chest pain. The pulse is usually weak, the blood pressure low, and the electrocardiogram (ECG) may show right ventricular strain. When rapid obstruction of 50% or more of the pulmonary vascular bed occurs, acute cor pulmonale (right-sided heart failure) may result because the right ventricle can no longer pump blood to the lungs. Death occurs in more than 60% of clients with massive emboli. Medium-sized emboli usually cause pleuritic chest pain, dyspnea, slight fever, and a productive cough with blood-streaked sputum. Tachycardia and pleural friction rub may be detected on physical examination. Small emboli frequently are undetected or produce vague transient symptoms, unless the client has a history of cardiopulmonary disease. These clients would respond even to small emboli that could result in severe cardiopulmonary compromise.

3. Discuss the most common clinical manifestations of PE. The severity of clinical manifestations of PE depends on the size of the emboli and the size and number of blood vessels occluded. *Anxiety* is an expected response to *ineffective breathing pattern* that occurs because the client has a sense of suffocation and inability to catch one's breath that accompanies pulmonary embolus, which is a strong physiologic stressor. *Unexplained dyspnea* is an acute response to the alteration in blood flow and oxygen to the lungs, which may be due to a medium-sized emboli, or is compounded by the level of anxiety, and also as a conscious awareness that breathing is needed to meet the metabolic demands of the body. *Tachypnea* occurs also due to the lack of oxygen, or as a compensatory action to the dyspnea. *Tachycardia* is also a compensatory response to the lack of blood flow, therefore, the heart beats faster in an attempt to increase blood flow to the lungs. Anxiety

and dyspnea are psychological stressors that cause the body's compensatory mechanisms to launch a fight-or-flight response. This information is relayed to the cardiac center in the medulla, and the sympathetic nervous system is stimulated to produce changes in the pulse.

4. **Discuss the complications of PE.** *Pulmonary infarction* (death of the lung tissue) will occur if the following factors are present: (1) occlusion of a large- or medium-sized pulmonary vessel (greater than 2 mm in diameter), (2) insufficient collateral blood flow from the bronchial circulation, or (3) preexisting lung disease. Infarction results in alveolar necrosis and hemorrhage, and if the infarct becomes infected, an abscess may develop. *Pulmonary hypertension* is another complication of PE that occurs when more than 50% of the area of the normal pulmonary bed is compromised. Pulmonary hypertension also results from hypoxemia. However, a single event of an embolus does not cause pulmonary hypertension unless it is massive, but recurrent small- or medium-sized emboli may result in chronic pulmonary hypertension. Pulmonary hypertension can eventually result in hypertrophy of the right ventricle, and depending on the degree of pulmonary hypertension and the rate of its development, death may result rapidly.

5. **Discuss diagnostic studies or serum labs used to confirm PE.** A *lung scan* (ventilation-perfusion scan) is the traditional screening test used for recurrent PE, to assess the natural history of the lesion and also to evaluate the effectiveness of therapy. It is a nuclear study that uses a radiopharmaceutical media injected IV or inhaled, after which scanning of the lungs is done to obtain views of the lungs and evaluate blood flow or perfusion (perfusion scan) and patency of the pulmonary airways or ventilation (ventilation scan). The results of the scan are compared with pulmonary function tests, chest X-ray, pulmonary angiography, and arterial blood gases. Nursing responsibilities include reinforcing with the client the length of time the study takes (30 minutes). The client is informed that a breathing mask may be used to administer the pharmaceutical agent or that the agent will be administered via intravenous line. The client will also be told that he or she will be expected to remain still during the procedure.

If the PE is suspected, a D-dimer testing may be recommended. D-dimer is a serum test that is used as a confirmatory test for altered coagulation stat. It assesses both thrombin and plasma activity. If the D-dimer level is elevated, a venogram (phlebogram) is done to look for DVT as the source for PE. If a DVT is located by the venogram, anticoagulant treatment should be initiated immediately. If the D-dimer level is elevated (above 500 ug/mL) but the venogram is normal, the client usually gets a lung scan.

If the lung scan is not conclusive, a pulmonary angiography is recommended to locate the clot and determine its size. Pulmonary angiogram uses an iodinated contrast medium that is injected into the pulmonary artery or a branch of the pulmonary vessel to locate the clot. The client is placed in a supine position and ECG machine leads are attached to the chest to identify dysrhythmias during the procedure. The procedure requires an informed consent and is done under sterile technique with a local anesthetic injected at the site of entry, then a small incision is made or a needle inserted. The catheter is inserted into the antecubital, femoral, brachial, or jugular vein and threaded into the inferior vena cava then into the right side of the heart under fluoroscope guidance. After the catheter enters the right ventricle, it is placed into the pulmonary artery, and the dye (medium) is injected. Serial films are taken during the injection of the dye to visualize pulmonary circulation. After the procedure is completed, the catheter is removed and a pressure dressing is applied to the site to prevent bleeding. After the procedure, nursing responsibilities include monitoring vital signs, monitoring site of entry for swelling, checking for signs of bleeding or hematoma, monitoring peripheral pulses of bilateral extremities, listening effectively for complaints of pain at the insertion site (discomfort may be a complaint). If client reports pain, nurse should question intensity and duration of pain. This should be reported to the health care provider appropriately, documenting the client's complaint.

The spiral (or helical) CT scan is a relatively new, noninvasive diagnostic test that can be used to diagnose PE. The benefits of the spiral CT is that it is able to continuously rotate while obtaining slices (images) and does not have to start and stop between each slice. This allows visualization of entire anatomic regions, such as the lungs. The data from the spiral CT can also be computer constructed to allow for a three-dimensional picture of the area being imaged and assist in emboli visualization.

6. What are common nursing diagnoses for clients with PE?

- Impaired gas exchange R/T altered pulmonary tissue perfusion
- Risk for injury, bleeding R/T pharmacologic therapy for PE
- Decreased cardiac output R/T acute pulmonary hypertension
- Deficient knowledge R/T condition, treatment, and health maintenance

The following are prescribed:

- Arterial blood gas (ABG) PRN
- Enoxaparin (Lovenox) 1mg/kg SC q12h
- Heparin sodium infusion 40,000 units in 1000 mL 0.9% normal saline at 40 mL/hr
- Warfarin sodium (Coumadin) 5 mg PO at 5 PM pending PT with INR
- Continuous pulse oximeter
- Continuous IV Dextrose 5% W in 0.45% NaCL at 75 mL/hr
- Serum labs: PT with INR, PTT daily
- Sequential compression bilateral devices for lower extremities

7. **What are the purposes for the prescribed orders?** *Arterial blood gas* readings provide close monitoring of the acid-base balance, respiratory status, and metabolic balance or imbalance and assess the adequacy of oxygenation. *Enoxaparin* prevents recurrence of PE and prophylaxis for DVT, which is a common cause of PE. It works by binding to a substance called antithrombin III, which turns off the three main activating factors: activated II, activated X, and activated IX. In doing so, it turns off the coagulation pathway and prevents clots from forming. It is a low-molecular-weight anticoagulant drug.

Heparin sodium infusion prevents excessive coagulation. It prevents thrombus formation by exerting direct effect on blood coagulation (clotting) through enhancement of the inhibitory actions of antithrombin III on activated II, activated IX, and activated X, thereby blocking the conversion of prothrombin to thrombin and fibrinogen to fibrin, which prevents the coagulation pathway from functioning.

Warfarin sodium is an oral anticoagulant that deters further extension of existing thrombi and prevents new clots from forming by indirectly interfering with blood clotting by depressing hepatic synthesis of vitamin K-dependent coagulation factors: II, VII, IX, and X.

Continuous pulse oximeter provides information regarding tissue perfusion and oxygen saturation in the periphery, identifies hemoglobin saturation, and alerts the nurse of desaturation before clinical signs develop. Results lower than 91%, and certainly 86%, constitute the need for immediate intervention. The *intravenous infusion* of 5% dextrose and 0.45% sodium chloride maintains hydration status and helps prevent venous stasis, due to the client's current immobile state.

The *PT with INR* provides information about the client's clotting status and guides Coumadin therapy. The therapeutic range is determined by an international normalized ratio. A therapeutic INR is considered to be 2.0–3.5. However, this range is disease specific, and therefore, the preferred INR for client's with pulmonary embolism is 3.0–4.0. The *PTT* evaluates clotting factors and is used to monitor heparin therapy. Clients receiving anticoagulant therapy should have a PTT value of 60–70 seconds and 1.5–2.5 times the control value in seconds. Both the PT with INR and the PTT are evaluated daily when Coumadin and heparin are to be administered on an ongoing basis.

The *sequential compression devices* to bilateral extremities help prevent DVT by providing intermittent compression to increase peripheral venous return and prevent venous stasis.

8. **What are the most common adverse reactions, drug-to-drug, drug-to-food/herbal interactions for the prescribed medications?** The most common adverse reactions of *enoxoparin* are bruising, bleeding, anemia, ecchymosis, and thrombocytopenia. Drug-to-drug interactions may occur with the simultaneous use of warfarin, aspirin, nonsteroidal anti-inflammatory agents (NSAIDs), dipyridamole, some penicillins, clopidogrel, ticlopidine, abciximab, eftifibatide, tirofiban, thrombolytics, and dextran, which alter platelet function and may increase the risk of hemorrhage. Drug-to-food/herbal interactions may occur with the simultaneous use of anise, arnica, chamomile, clove, garlic, ginger, gingko, feverfew, horse chestnut, and Panax ginseng, which may increase risk for bleeding. The most common adverse reactions of *heparin therapy* are bleeding, which may be uncontrolled; bruising; epistaxis; tarry stools; vasospastic reactions resulting in painful ischemic extremity; anemia; and transient thrombocytopenia. Drug-to-drug interactions may occur with the simultaneous use of oral anticoagulants, aspirin, adrenocortico steroids, cefamandole, cefoperazone, cefotetan, moxalactam, dextran, penicillins, dipyridamole, glycooprotein GPIIb/IIIa receptor antagonists, tirofiban, ticlopidine, phenylbutazone, hydroxychloroquine, indomethacin, detorolac, plicamycin, probenecid, alteplase, anistreplase, streptokinase, thyroid agents, valproic acid, and NSAIDS, which will increase the risk of bleeding. The simultaneous use of nitroglycerin infusion may decrease anticoagulant activity, and also the effects of protamine sulfate, which is the antidote for heparin toxicity. Antihistamines, digoxin, nicotine, and tetracyclines inhibit the effects of heparin. There are no clinically significant drug-to-food interactions established. Drug-to-herbal interactions may occur with the simultaneous use of anise, arnica, chamomile, clove, dong quai, feverfew, gingko, ginger, and valerian, which may potentiate bleeding. A common adverse reaction of *warfarin sodium* is prolonged clotting time producing bruising and increased risk for uncontrolled bleeding. Drug-to-drug interactions may occur with the simultaneous use of heparin, which will enhance the effects of warfarin and increase bleeding. The simultaneous use of acetaminophen, aminoglycoside antibiotics, amiodarone, androgens, beta-adrenergic blocking agents, bromeliad, capecitabine, celecoxib, cephalosporins, chloral hydrate, chloramphenicol, cimetidine, clarithromycin, clofibrate, contrast media containing iodine, corticosteroids, cyclophosphamide, dextrothyroxine, diflunisal, erythromycin, fluconazole, gemfibrozil, glucagons, hydantoins, oral hypoglycemics, ifosfamide, indomethacin, isoniazid, itraconazole, ketoconazole, loop diuretics, lovastatin, metronidazole, miconazole, morizine, nalidixic acid, NSAIDs, omeprazole, penicillins, propafenone, propoxyphene, quinidine, quinolones, streptokinase, sulfamethoxazole/trimethoprim, sulfinpyrazone, sulfonamides, sulindac, tamoxifen, tetracyclines, thioamines, thyroid hormones, and urokinase also enhance bleeding tendencies. Agents that decrease the effects of warfarin include alcohol use (chronic), aminoglutethimide, barbiturates, carbamazepine, cholestyramine, oral contraceptives, dicloxacillin, estrogens, etretinate, glutethimide, griseofulvin, nafcillin, nevirapine, rifampin, ritonavir, spirolactone, sucralfate, thiazide diuretics, thiopurines, and trazodone. Drug-to-food interactions may occur with the simultaneous use of vitamins A, C, and E, which enhance warfarin's effects, and vitamin K, which is the antidote for warfarin toxicity. Drug-to-herbal interactions may occur with the simultaneous use of capsicum, celery, chamomile, cinchona bark, clove, devil's claw, dong quai, Echinacea, evening primrose oil, fenugreek, feverfew, garlic, ginseng panax, ginger, gingko, grapeseed abstract, horse chestnut, licorice root, passion flower, herb, tumeric, and willow bark (which may increase the risk of bleeding), many of which act by decreasing platelet aggregation. The simultaneous use of avocado, ginseng, green tea, and St. John's Wort may decrease the effectiveness of *warfarin.*

9. Discuss three surgical procedures a health care provider may anticipate for a client with multiple large pulmonary emboli if fibrinolytic therapy is contraindicated. The two surgical procedures are *balloon embolectomy, surgical embolectomy,* and an *inferior vena cava interruption.* A *balloon embolectomy* is an invasive procedure that requires a signed consent. During the procedure, a deflated balloon catheter is passed in the vessel beyond the embolus. The balloon is then inflated, and the embolus is removed. A *surgical embolectomy* involves an incision into an artery for the removal of an embolus. It is usually performed as an emergency management intervention. Most embolus begins in the lower extremities and travel to other areas of the body, lodging in areas such as the aorta, the common carotid arteries, or the pulmonary arteries. Before surgery, heparin may be administered and an arteriogram used to identify the affected artery. After surgery, blood pressure is maintained close to the preoperative baseline, since a decrease in blood pressure may predispose the client to a new clot formation. An *inferior venae cava interruption* is the insertion of an umbrellalike filter (Greenfield filter) into the inferior cava to trap large emboli while at the same time allowing continued blood flow. This procedure is used when venous thrombosis is recurrent and anticoagulant therapy is contraindicated. The filter is inserted under fluoroscopy with local anesthesia. After the procedure, the client's vital signs and peripheral pulses are checked for deviations, and documenting and reporting should be included in the focus for postprocedure care.

10. Discuss client education for someone being discharged following successful treatment for a PE. The lifestyle changes that can help reduce the risk for PE include cessation of smoking. Prolonged cigarette smoking causes vasoconstriction of blood vessels, which eventually impairs blood flow, resulting in thrombus formation. To reduce the risk associated with long periods of immobility and to lessen the risk of venous stasis, the client should stop every one to two hours during long automobile trips for a brief stretch and

walk; get up every few hours and do leg exercises during long air flights; avoid crossing the legs; do regular exercises, such as walking; and avoid using tight-fitted elastic stockings or hose that bind around the knee or thigh.

References

Black, J. M and Hawks, J. H. (2005). *Medical-Surgical Nursing: Clinical Management for Positive Outcomes* (7th ed.). Philadelphia: W. B. Saunders.

Broyles, B. E. (2005). *Medical-Surgical Nursing Clinical Companion.* Durham, NC: Carolina Academic Press.

Gahart, B. L. and Nazareno, A. R. (2005). *2005 Intraveneous Medications.* St. Louis: Elsevier Mosby.

Harkreader, H. and Hogan, M. A. (2004). *Fundamentals of Nursing: Caring and Clinical Judgment* (2nd ed.). Philadelphia: W. B. Saunders.

Huether, S. E. and McCance, K. L. (2004). *Understanding Pathophysiology* (3rd ed.). St. Louis: Mosby.

Ignatavicius, D. D. and Workman, M. L. (2006). *Medical-Surgical Nursing across the Health Care Continuum* (5th ed.). Philadelphia: W. B. Saunders.

Koschel, M. J. (2004). "Pulmonary Embolism: Quick Diagnosis Can Save a Patient's Life." *American Journal of Nursing* 104(6): 46–50.

Skidmore-Roth, L. (2006). *Mosby's Handbook of Herbs and Natural Supplements* (3rd ed.). St. Louis: Mosby.

Spratto, G. R. and Woods, A. L. (2005). *2005 Edition: PDR Nurse's Drug Handbook.* Clifton Park, NY: Thomson Delmar Learning.

CASE STUDY 4

Systemic Lupus Erythematosus

GENDER

F

AGE

40

SETTING

Hospital

ETHNICITY/CULTURE

- Black American/West Indian

PREEXISTING CONDITIONS

- Community-acquired pneumonia
- Pulmonary tuberculosis

COEXISTING CONDITIONS

- Renal failure

LIFESTYLE

- RN/nurse educator

COMMUNICATION

DISABILITY

SOCIOECONOMIC STATUS

- Middle

SPIRITUAL/RELIGIOUS

- Seventh Day Adventist

PHARMACOLOGIC

- Folic acid (Apo-Folic)

- Topical hydrocortisone
- Ibuprofen (Motrin)
- Methotrexate (Rheumatrex Dose Pack)
- Methylprednisolone sodium succinate (Solu-Medrol)
- Misoprostol (Cytotec)
- Prednisone (Deltasone)
- Hydroxychloroquine sulfate (Plaquenil)

PSYCHOSOCIAL

- Anxiety
- Depression
- Fear

LEGAL

- Financial support for ongoing home health care

ETHICAL

- Persons who worked for years but are now incapacitated should have optimum health benefits to offset medical costs.

ALTERNATIVE THERAPY

- Homeopathic medicine

PRIORITIZATION

- Relieve discomfort
- Decrease immune complexes in coronary vessels
- Maintenance of skin integrity

DELEGATION

- RN
- Client education

DIFFICULT

THE RESPIRATORY AND IMMUNE SYSTEMS

Level of difficulty: Difficult

Overview: This case involves a thorough assessment of all systems. It involves monitoring temperature for indication of pending exacerbation and questioning the client about skin changes, specifically sensitivity to sunlight; complaints of generalized weakness; and weight loss. It involves assessing for signs of renal involvement and central nervous system effects, which could include psychosis and seizures. The nurse must use critical-thinking skills to appropriately prioritize care in a busy emergency department (ED) of a large urban environment.

Client Profile

Mrs. N is a 40-year-old divorced registered nurse, administrative nursing supervisor, and nurse educator who has been active with daily activities and her professional assignments for several years. Mrs. N was divorced five years ago and, soon after, developed primary hypertension.

Case Study

Mrs. N is under the care of her family health care provider for the hypertension, which fluctuated from stabilized to very high levels. Mrs. N's health gradually deteriorated, and she returned home to her native island for a reprieve. After three months, she returned to the United States and was employed by a nursing school, where she was a full-time clinical instructor. During a clinical rotation, Mrs. N reported "not feeling her usual self" and was accompanied to the agency's emergency department (ED), where she was admitted for overnight observation. On initial history and data gather, she reports a history of community-acquired pneumonia (CAP) and pulmonary tuberculosis. On assessment, Mrs. N manifests butterfly rash across the cheeks and bridge of the nose, erythematous fingertip lesions. She complains of feeling tired regardless of decrease in daily activities, anorexia, malaise, and weight loss. Vital signs on admission are:

Blood pressure: 120/84
Pulse: 106
Respirations: 14
Temperature: 100° F

A health care provider sees the client, and the history and physical examination are done. Magnetic resonance imaging (MRI) of the hip joints is negative, and MRI of the brain found no characteristic abnormalities. Blood specimens are drawn and sent for anti-DNA antibody and anti-phospholipid antibodies titer, antinuclear antibodies level, complement levels C_3 and C_4, complete blood count, blood urea nitrogen (BUN), and creatinine. The results of the tests are:

Anti-DNA antibody and antiphospholipid: reveal high titers
Antinuclear antibody titer: increased above 50
Complement C_3: 60 mg/dL
Complement C_4: 8 mg/dL
Complete blood count: pantocytopenia (a decrease in all cells)
Blood urea nitrogen (BUN): 30 mg/dL
Creatinine: 2.6 mg/dL

After the laboratory results are reviewed by a rheumatologist, the diagnosis of systemic lupus erythematosus (SLE) is confirmed and discussed with the multidisciplinary team. The confirmation and plan of care is discussed with the client, who agreed with the plan of care.

Questions

1. Discuss the incidence, etiology, risk factors, and pathophysiology of systemic lupus erythematosus (SLE).

2. Discuss clinical manifestations of SLE.

3. Discuss systemic manifestations of SLE.

4. Discuss the diagnostic findings of SLE.

5. Discuss the medical management of SLE.

6. What are the purposes for the prescribed orders?

7. What are the most common adverse reactions, drug-to-drug, drug-to-food/herbal interactions of the prescribed medications?

8. Discuss pericardial tamponade, a complication of SLE.

9. Discuss the main goals of care for the client with SLE.

10. Discuss client education for SLE.

Questions and Suggested Answers

1. Discuss the incidence, etiology, risk factors, and pathophysiology of SLE. SLE occurs most commonly in younger women between the ages of 15 and 40 years. It is almost 10 times more common in women than in men. It is more common in black women. It has a familial tendency, and when one twin has the disease, the other twin has a 60–70% chance of acquiring it. It is an autoimmune disease involving diffuse inflammatory changes of the vascular and connective tissue.

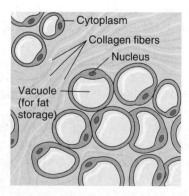

Connective tissue is found almost everywhere within the body: bones, cartilage, mucous membranes, muscles, nerves, skin, and all internal organs.

Although the exact cause is not known, causes of disease exacerbation have been identified and include sunlight and other forms of ultraviolet light, physical and emotional stress, and pregnancy. There is a form of drug-induced SLE associated with adverse reactions to some drugs, including hydralazine (Apresoline), and other drugs such as phenytoin (Dilantin) and phenobarbital are known to produce an SLE-like syndrome. The drug-induced problems resolve when the drugs are discontinued. SLE is a chronic, progressive, systemic inflammatory connective tissue disease that develops insidiously. It produces inflammatory, biochemical, and structural changes in the vascular and connective tissue as well as in the viscera, joints, fascia, tendons, and bursae. It is characterized by remissions and exacerbation. Several abnormal serum protein factors and antinuclear antibodies (ANA) may be found with SLE that suggest an autoimmune mechanism is occurring. The ANA mainly affect the deoxyribonucleic acid (DNA) within the cell nuclei, leading to the formation of immune complexes in serum and organ tissues. Characteristic histologic findings are lupus erythematosus (LE) cells and extracellular masses called hematoxylin bodies. However, LE cells may be found in many diseases and may or may not be demonstrated with SLE. Most clients with SLE have a mild to moderate, normochromic anemia, and the ESR is usually elevated. A mild leukopenia is often present, and serum globulins may be increased. There is some degree of kidney involvement causing progressive changes within the glomeruli in most clients, and eventually with progression, the client develops nephritis and the end result being renal failure.

2. **Discuss clinical manifestations of SLE.** General manifestations include fatigue, malaise, and episodic fever. Musculoskeletal manifestations include arthralgia, arthritis, morning stiffness, and joint deformities. Integumentary manifestations include photosensitivity, butterfly rash, discoid lesions of skin and mucous membranes, alopecia, and telangiectasia. Neurologic manifestations include neuropathy, stroke, headache, and seizure. Pulmonary manifestations include cough, dyspnea, pleurisy, and pneumonitis. Cardiovascular manifestations include pericardial effusion, myocarditis, coronary artery disease, valvular disease, thrombophlebitis, Raynaud's phenomenon, and vasculitis. Hematologic manifestations include anemia, leukopenia, thrombocytopenia, lymphadenopathy, splenomegaly, and antibodies to clotting factors. Renal manifestations include nephritis, glomerulonephritis, and urinary tract infection. Gastrointestinal (GI) manifestations include dysphagia, nausea, vomiting, pancreatitis, and elevated liver function tests. Psychiatric manifestations include anxiety, depression, and psychosis.

3. **Discuss systemic manifestations of SLE.** Involvement of the musculoskeletal system is seen with arthralgia and arthritis (synovitis) is a common

presenting feature of SLE. Joint swelling, tenderness, and pain on movement are also common and frequently accompanied by morning stiffness. Skin reactions involve subacute cutaneous lupus erythematosus, which involves papulosquamous or annular polycyclicthematous papules or plaques and scaling, and cause scarring and pigmentation changes. The most familiar skin manifestation is an acute cutaneous lesion consisting of a butterfly-shaped rash across the bridge of the nose and cheeks. There are erythematous rashes on the skin with cutaneous erythematous plaques observed on the scalp, face, or neck. Areas of hyperpigmentation or depigmentation may be evident depending on the phase of the disease. The scalp is inspected for alopecia, and the mouth and throat for ulcerations reflecting gastrointestinal involvement. Papular, erythematous, and purpuric lesions developing on the fingertips, elbows, toes, and extensor surfaces of the forearms or lateral sides of the hand may become necrotic, suggesting vascular involvement. Oral ulcers may involve the buccal mucosa or the hard palate. Pericarditis is the most common cardiac manifestation, and women with SLE are at risk for atherosclerosis. There is pericardial friction rub, possibly associated with myocarditis and pleural effusion. The pleural effusions and infiltrations are evidenced by abnormal lung sounds. Depression and psychosis are common. Hematuria may be found on urinalysis.

4. **Discuss the diagnostic findings of SLE.** No single laboratory test confirms SLE; rather, blood testing reveals moderate to severe anemia, thrombocytopenia, leukocytosis, or leucopenia, and positive antinuclear antibodies.

5. **Discuss the medical management of SLE.** Medical management involves treating both acute and chronic SLE. Acute disease requires interventions directed at controlling increased disease activity or exacerbations that may involve any organ system. Management of chronic condition involves periodic monitoring and recognition of clinical changes, and modification of therapy.

The following are prescribed:

- Topical hydrocortisone 2.5% ointment, liberal amount to the face daily
- Ibuprofen (Motrin) 800 mg PO two times per day
- Misoprostol (Cytotec) 200 mcg PO daily
- Methylprednisolone sodium succinate (Solu-Medrol) 50 mg q6h IV × one week
- Prednisone (Deltasone) 15 mg PO daily
- Methotrexate (Rheumatrex) 7.5 mg PO weekly
- Folic acid (Apo-Folic) 0.4 mg PO daily
- Hydroxychloroquine sulfate (Plaquenil) 10 mg PO daily

6. **What are the purposes for the prescribed orders?** *Topical hydrocortisone* to the face daily helps reduce inflammation and promotes fading of the skin lesions. It stabilizes the epidermal lysosomes in the skin and protects it

from the physiological trauma caused by the disease process. *Ibuprofen* is a nonsteroidal anti-inflammatory agent that helps to prevent thrombosis by decreasing or preventing platelet aggregation, which enhances systemic circulation, and prevents venous thrombosis. It also is beneficial for the mild polyarthralgia or polyarthritis that usually occurs with SLE. *Misoprostol* is a prostaglandin that minimizes the GI GI effects of ibuprofen. It does this by inhibiting basal and nocturnal gastric acid secretion and acid secretion in response to a variety of stimuli such as the consumption of aspirin. *Methylprednisolone sodium succinate* is a glucocorticoid used to abruptly stop the flare up of SLE, allowing the client to stay on a low-maintenance dose of steroid such as prednisone. It does this by suppressing inflammation and the normal immune response. *Prednisone* also is a glucocorticoid that slows the inflammatory process by suppressing inflammation and the normal immune response. *Methotrexate* is an antimetabolite antineoplastic agent that maintains remission of the disease process by blocking folic acid synthesis participation in nucleic acid synthesis, which slows the inflammatory process, and helps with remission. *Folic acid* is classified as a vitamin B complex agent that counteracts some of the adverse effects of methotrexate (e.g., aplastic anemia, leukopenia, thrombocytopenia). It does this by stimulating the production of red blood cells (RBCs), white blood cells (WBCs), and platelets. *Hydroxychloroquine sulfate* is an antirheumatic agent that reduces the inflammatory response and, therefore, decreases the frequency of attacks. It reduces the inflammatory response by inhibiting the replication and transcription of DNA and RNA synthesis, and decreases the formation of the immune complexes that aggravate the disease process.

7. **What are the most common adverse reactions, drug-to-drug, drug-to-food/herbal interactions of the prescribed medications?** There are no clinically significant common adverse reactions, drug-to-drug, and drug-to-food interactions established for topical corticosteroid (i.e., *hydrocortisone*). The most common adverse reactions of *ibuprofen* are nausea, vomiting, heartburn, and stomach pains. With *ibuprofen*, drug-to-drug interactions may occur with the concurrent use of furosemide causing a decreased diuretic effect because of decreased renal prostaglandin synthesis. Use with lithium increases plasma lithium levels resulting in increased risk of lithium toxicity. Ibuprofen decreases the effects of antihypertensives and thiazide diuretics, and if used with aspirin, its action is decreased. With simultaneous use of cefamandole, cefotetan, cefopenazone, valporic acid, thrombolytics, antiplatelets, and warfarin, ibuprofen may increase risk of bleeding. Increased possibility of blood dyscrasias may occur when used with antineoplastics or radiation therapy. *Ibuprofen* may increase the risk of toxicity when used with digoxin, cyclosporine, probenecid, and oral anticoagulants

and may increase the risk of hypoglycemia when used with oral hypoglycemics or insulin. When used concurrently with arnica, chamomile, clove, dong quai, fenugreek, feverfew, garlic, ginger, gingko, and ginseng, the client is at greater risk of bleeding. No clinically significant drug-to-food interactions are established, although ibuprofen should be taken with food to decrease GI symptoms. The most common adverse reactions of *misoprostol* are diarrhea and abdominal pain. With *misoprostol* drug-to-drug interactions may occur with the simultaneous use of magnesium containing antacids, which may increase diarrhea. There are no clinically significant drug-to-food/herbal interactions established except that absorption of misoprostol is decreased when taken with food. The most common adverse reactions of **methylprednisone sodium succinate** are depression, euphoria, hypertension, nausea, decreased wound healing, ecchymoses, fragility, hirsutism, petechiae, adrenal suppression, muscle wasting, osteoporosis, and cushingoid appearance. Drug-to-drug interactions may occur with the simultaneous use of cholestyramine, colestipol, barbiturates, phenytoin, theophylline, and rifampin, which increase *methylprednisolone sodium succinate* metabolism, requiring increased dosage of *methylprednisolone*. It decreases the effects of anticoagulants, anticonvulsants, antidiabetic agents, ambenonium, neostigmine, isoniazid, toxoids, vaccines, anticholinesterases, salicylates, and somatrem. Increased side effects of *methylprednisolone sodium succinate* occur with the simultaneous use of alcohol, salicylates, indomethacin, amphotericin B, digoxin, cyclosporine, neostigmine, pyridostigmine, and diuretics may increase potassium loss. Potassium deficiency may result with the simultaneous use of *methylprednisolone sodium succinate* and aloe, buckthorn, rhubarb, cascara sagrada, buckthorn, rhubarb root, and senna may cause severe muscle weakness in clients with myasthenia gravis. Other agents that increase the action of *methylprednisolone* include salicylates, estrogens, indomethacin, oral contraceptives, itraconazole, ritonavir, indinavir, saquinavir, erythromycin, ketoconazole, and macrolide antibiotics. The simultaneous use of grapefruit juice may increase the serum levels. The most common adverse effects of *methotrexate* include bone marrow suppression, hepatotoxicity, increased uric acid, acne, ecchymoses, leukoencephalopathy, and fetal death if used during pregnancy. With *methotrexate* drug-to-drug interactions may occur with the simultaneous use of salicylates, sulfa drugs, other antineoplastic agents, radiation, alcohol, probenecid, nonsteroidal anti-inflammatory agents (NSAIDs), phenylbutazone, theophylline, and penicillins, resulting in increased toxicity. *Methotrexate* may decrease the effects of digoxin, vaccines, phenytoin, and fosphenytoin. If used concurrently with oral anticoagulants there is an increased risk of hypoprothrombinemia. Folic acid supplements may decrease methotrexate effects. The most common adverse reactions of *prednisone* are (similar to methylprednisone sodium succinate) depression, euphoria, hypertension, nausea, decreased wound healing, ecchymoses, fragility, hirsutism, petechiae, adrenal suppression, muscle wasting, osteoporosis, and cushingoid appearance. With the simultaneous use of *prednisone* and cholestyramine, colestipol, barbiturates, rifampin, phenytoin, and theophylline, the action of prednisone may be decreased. Decreased effects of anticoagulants, anticonvulsants, oral hypoglycemics and insulin, ambenonium, neostigmine, isoniazid, vaccines, anticholinesterases, salicylates, and somatrem may be caused by *prednisone*. Increase in the side effects of prednisone may occur with the concurrent use of alcohol, salicylates, indomethacin, amphotericin B, digoxin, cyclosporine, and diuretics. Other agents that increase the action of *prednisone* include salicylates, estrogens, indomethacin, oral contraceptives, ketoconazole, and macrolide antibiotics. The only clinically significant adverse effects associated with *folic acid* are bronchospasm and flushing of the skin. With *folic acid* drug-to-drug interactions are rare but include methotrexate; sulfonamides; and sulfasalazine, which decrease folate levels and estrogens; hydantoins; carbamazepine; and glucocorticoids that increase the need for folic acid. There are no clinically significant drug-to-food/herbal interactions established. The most common adverse reaction of *hydroxychloroquine sulfate* is blurred vision, corneal changes, retinopathy, difficulty focusing, photophobia, seizures, and hypotension. Drug-to-drug interactions may occur with the simultaneous use of *hydroxychloroquine* and aluminum and magnesium containing antacids and laxatives, which decrease *hydroxychloroquine* absorption. *Hydroxychloroquine* increases serum levels of digoxin, increasing the risk of toxicity. Use with rabies vaccine may cause an increased antibody titer. There are no clinically significant drug-to-food/herbal interactions established.

8. **Discuss pericardial tamponade, a complication of SLE.** Clients with SLE often develop pericarditis caused by either bacterial or viral infections. Acute pericarditis has exudate that may be serous, purulent, or hemorrhagic. If the exudate accumulates in the pericardial sac, pericardial tamponade develops, and without prompt treatment, shock and death can result. Pericardial tamponade is a cardiac emergency because the accumulated fluid restricts diastolic ventricular filling, and the end result is the compression of the heart and the restricting of blood low in and out of the ventricles. Large or rapidly accumulating effusions raise the intrapericardial pressure to a point at which venous blood cannot flow into the heart, which decreases ventricular filling, resulting in an increase in venous pressure and fall in cardiac output and arterial blood pressure. Tachycardia is initially present as the heart compensates by beating rapidly, but tachycardia cannot sustain the cardiac output for very long, therefore prompt intervention is needed to prevent shock and death. The emergency intervention of choice is pericardiocentesis, which involves aspirating the

fluid from the pericardial sac. Nursing care before the procedure includes withholding anticoagulant medications and aspirin as ordered, having the client void, taking and recording vital signs, and administering premedication as ordered. During the procedure the client is observed for respiratory or cardiac distress. Nursing care after the procedure includes assisting the client to a position of comfort, resuming foods or fluids withheld before the test. Continue intravenous fluids until vital signs are stable and the client is able to resume normal fluid intake. Assess the puncture site for bleeding, hematoma formation, and inflammation each time vital signs are taken and daily thereafter for several days. Administer antibiotic specific to the causative agent and anti-inflammatory drugs to reduce the inflammatory response.

9. Discuss the main goals of care for the client with SLE. *Preservation of organ function* (e.g., integumentary): the client will understand the importance of avoiding exposure to sun and ultraviolet light by protecting self with sunscreen and clothing. Given the increased risk for cardiovascular disease, including hypertension and atherosclerosis, the client will understand the importance of continuing with prescribed medications and dietary regimen as shared by a registered dietitian. *Prevention of organ failure* (e.g., renal and cardiac): the client will understand the need for routine periodic screenings as well as health promotion activities and follow-up care with a health care provider.

10. Discuss client education for SLE. The client should take hydroxychloroquine sulfate with food or a light snack to avoid stomach discomfort. Report any form of blurred vision or headache, because the drug may cause damage to areas of the eyes. The client should have an eye examination every six to twelve months so that changes can be detected and treated immediately. If any unusual changes occur with the eyes, the drug should be stopped and the primary health care provider or a hospital ED should be contacted immediately. The client should use sun-blocking agent with a sun protection factor (SPF) to help protect skin from sun exposure; inspect the skin daily for open areas and rashes; apply lotion to skin liberally; and wear a large-brimmed hat, long sleeves, and long pants when in the sun.

References

Broyles, B. E. (2005). *Medical-Surgical Nursing Clinical Companion*. Durham, NC: Carolina Academic Press.

Corbet, J. V. (2004). *Laboratory Tests and Diagnostic Procedures with Nursing Diagnoses* (6th ed.). Upper Saddle River, NJ: Prentice Hall.

Gahart, B. L. and Nazareno, A. R. (2005). *2005 Intravenous Medications*. St. Louis: Elsevier Mosby.

Guyton, A. C. and Hall, J. E. (2006). *Textbook of Medical Physiology* (11th ed.). Philadelphia: W. B. Saunders.

Heitz, U. and Horne, M. M. (2005). *Mosby's Pocket Guide Series: Fluid, Electrolyte and Acid-Base Balance* (5th ed.). St. Louis: Mosby.

Huether, S. E. and McCance, K. L. (2004). *Understanding Pathophysiology* (3rd ed.). St. Louis: Mosby.

Ignatavicius, D. D. and Workman, M. L. (2006). *Medical-Surgical Nursing across the Health Care Continuum* (5th ed.). Philadelphia: W. B. Saunders.

Petri, M. (June 1998). "Treatment of Systemic Lupus Erythematosus: An Update." *American Family Physician* 57(11): 2753–2762. Available at www.aafp.org/afp/980600ap/petri.html

Spratto, G. R. and Woods, A. L. (2005). *2005 Edition: PDR Nurse's Drug Handbook*. Clifton Park, NY: Thomson Delmar Learning.

www.medicinet.com (December 2005). Systemic Lupus Erythematosus.

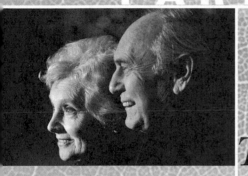

PART THREE

The Cardiovascular and Lymphatic Systems

Buerger's Disease
(Thromboangiitis Obliterans)

GENDER

M

AGE

32

SETTING

- Health care provider's office

ETHNICITY/CULTURE

- Asian/Philippines

PREEXISTING CONDITIONS

COEXISTING CONDITIONS

- Digital rest pain

LIFESTYLE

- College student

COMMUNICATION

- English and Tagalo

DISABILITY

- Decrease in ambulatory status

SOCIOECONOMIC STATUS

- Low

SPIRITUAL/RELIGIOUS

- Catholic
- Belief that God gives will to bear pain

PHARMACOLOGIC

- Oxycodone HcL (Roxicodone)
- Ibuprofen (Motrin)
- Prednisone (Deltasone)
- Prazosin HcL (Minipress)
- Pentoxifylline (Trental)

PSYCHOSOCIAL

- Grief
- Fear
- Anxiety

LEGAL

- Lack of insurance should not negate optimum health care.

ETHICAL

- Pain is an objective symptom. The client's report of pain should be appropriately evaluated and treated.

ALTERNATIVE THERAPY

- Regular exercise
- Ginseng

PRIORITIZATION

- Relieve pain

DELEGATION

- RN
- CNA
- Client education

MODERATE

THE CARDIOVASCULAR AND LYMPHATIC SYSTEMS

Level of difficulty: Moderate

Overview: This case involves a thorough assessment of the client's condition including any drug or herbals he is currently taking. It also involves critical history and physical examination to gather appropriate data for nursing diagnosis and implementation. The certified nursing assistant can take height, weight, and vital signs and report complaints of pain or discomfort to the nurse.

Client Profile

Mr. Y is a 34-year-old student enrolled in a respiratory therapy program. He is seen at the health care provider's office for complaints of aching pain in the lower extremities while at rest. He tells the health care provider during the health history that he smoked three packs of cigarette a day for ten years but has presently decreased the number of packs of cigarettes smoked per day to two, with the hope he will gradually "kick" the smoking habit.

Case Study

On physical assessment his peripheral pulses of the lower extremities are at times fleeting and at times absent. In the dependent position, the extremities are cool and red. His vital signs are:

Blood pressure: 110/80
Pulse: 78
Respirations: 18
Temperature: 98.6° F

Serum labs:

White blood cell (WBC) count: 8,000/mm^3
Hematocrit (Hct): 37%
Hemoglobin (Hgb): 15 mg/dL

Diagnostic tests are scheduled by the nurse at the health care provider's office, and Mr. Y is given the dates for various tests. Mr. Y returns for the diagnostic tests as scheduled. The arteriogram of the lower extremities reveals multiple sequential occlusions in the smaller arteries of the forearm, hands, and feet. The plethysmographic studies show slight decrease in pressure of the fingers and toes, and ankle-brachial index is 0.7 in bilateral legs. After the diagnostic tests and laboratory data are reviewed, a diagnosis of Buerger's disease is confirmed and discussed with Mr. Y.

Questions

1. Discuss the incidence, prevalence, risk factors, and pathophysiology of Buerger's disease.

2. Discuss gerontologic considerations of Buerger's disease.

3. Discuss clinical manifestations of Buerger's disease.

4. Discuss assessment and diagnostic findings of Buerger's disease.

5. What are the purposes for the prescribed orders?

6. What are the most common adverse reactions, drug-to-drug, drug-to-food/herbal interactions for the prescribed medications?

7. Discuss medical and nursing management of complications of Buerger's disease.

8. Discuss surgical management of complications of Buerger's disease.

9. Discuss Buerger-Allen exercise.

10. Discuss client education for Buerger's disease.

Questions and Suggested Answers

1. **Discuss the incidence, prevalence, risk factors, and pathophysiology of Buerger's disease.** Buerger's disease has been reported in all races and in many areas of the world. It occurs most often in men between the ages of 20 and 35 years. The predominant cause is cigarette smoking or chewing of tobacco. It is generally bilateral, with the lower extremities affected, but arteries in the upper extremities or viscera can also be involved.

2. **Discuss gerontologic considerations of Buerger's disease.** Although this condition is different from atherosclerosis, Buerger's disease in older persons may also be followed by atherosclerosis of the larger vessels after involvement of the smaller vessels. The person's ability to walk may be severely limited, and they are at higher risk for nonhealing wounds because of impaired circulation.

3. **Discuss clinical manifestations of Buerger's disease.** Pain is the outstanding symptom, and intermittent claudication is a common problem that occurs in almost all clients at some stage of the disease. Complaints of foot cramps, especially of the arch (instep claudication), after exercise is reported. Cold sensitivity of the hands is also reported, and digital rest pain is constant, and the characteristics of the pain do not change between activity and rest. Physical signs include intense rubor (reddish blue discoloration) of the foot and absence of the pedal pulse but with normal femoral and popliteal pulses. Radial and ulnar artery pulses are absent or diminished, and various types of paresthesia may develop. As the disease progresses, definite redness or cyanosis of the part appears when the extremity is in a dependent position. Color changes may progress to ulceration, and ulceration with gangrene eventually occurs.

4. **Discuss assessment and diagnostic findings of Buerger's disease.** The diagnosis is commonly based on a physical finding of peripheral ischemia, often in association with migratory superficial phlebitis. Segmental limb blood pressures are taken to demonstrate the distal location of the lesions or occlusions. Duplex ultrasonography is used to document patency of the proximal vessels and to visualize the extent of distal disease. Contrast angiography is performed to demonstrate the diseased portion of the anatomy.

The following are prescribed:

- Oxycodone (Roxicodone) 5–10 mg PO q4h PRN pain
- Ibuprofen (Motrin) 800 mg PO q8h PRN pain
- Prednisone (Deltasone) 10 mg PO q6h
- Prazosin HcL (Minipress) 2 mg PO two times per day
- Pentoxifylline (Trental) 400 mg PO three times per day

5. What are the purposes for the prescribed orders? *Oxycodone* is an opiate analgesic prescribed to treat moderate to severe pain by depressing the perception of pain in the central nervous system. *Ibuprofen* is a nonsteroidal anti-inflammatory agent used to decrease pain by interfering with Cox-1 and Cox-2 prostaglandins. *Prednisone* is a glucocorticoid prescribed to decrease inflammation by interfering with the body's inflammatory process. *Prazosine HcL* is an alpha-1 adrenergic blocking antihypertensive prescribed because of its action in dilating arterioles and veins, decreasing total peripheral resistance and increasing circulation to the periphery to decrease intermittent claudication. *Pentoxifylline* is a hemorrheologic agent that acts by decreasing blood viscosity and stimulating prostacyclin (a prostaglandin) formation that increases red blood cell flexibility, improves peripheral blood flow, reduces tissue hypoxia, and decreases pain. It also reduces platelet aggregation interrupting the vicious cycle of tissue hypoxia, sludging and stasis of capillary blood flow, and reduced oxygen delivery to ischemic cells.

6. What are the most common adverse reactions, drug-to-drug, drug-to-food/herbal interactions of the prescribed medications? The most common adverse effect of *oxycodone HcL* is constipation. Other adverse effects include drowsiness, dizziness, euphoria, and fatigue. Drug-to-drug interactions may occur with the simultaneous use of *oxycodone HcL* and any other central nervous system (CNS) depressant including barbiturates, hydantoins, sedative-hypnotics, and additional opioid analgesics resulting in increased sedation. Use with protease inhibitors increases CNS depression and risk of respiratory depression. No clinically significant drug-to-food interactions have been established, however any herbals that cause CNS depression will increase the sedative effects of oxycodone. The most common adverse effect of *ibuprofen* is gastrointestinal (GI) distress. With *ibuprofen* drug-to-drug interactions may occur with the concurrent use of furosemide causing a decreased diuretic effect because of decreased renal prostaglandin synthesis. Use with lithium increases plasma lithium levels resulting in increased risk of lithium toxicity. Ibuprofen decreases the effects of antihypertensives and thiazide diuretics, and if used with aspirin, ibuprofen's action is decreased. With simultaneous use of cefamandole, cefotetan, cefopenazone, valporic acid, thrombolytics, antiplatelets, and warfarin, ibuprofen may increase risk of bleeding. Increased possibility of blood dyscrasias may occur when used with antineoplastics or radiation therapy. Ibuprofen may increase the risk of toxicity when used with digoxin, cyclosporine, probenecid, and oral anticoagulants and may increase the risk of hypoglycemia when used with oral hypoglycemics or insulin. When used concurrently with arnica, chamomile, clove, dong quai, fenugreek, feverfew, garlic, ginger, gingko, and ginseng, the client is at greater risk of bleeding. No clinically significant drug-to-food interactions are established, although ibuprofen should be taken with food to decrease GI symptoms. The most common adverse effects of *prednisone* are fluid retention, delayed wound healing, mood changes, flushing, headache, thrombocytopenia, fractures, and osteoporosis. Drug-to-drug interactions may occur with the simultaneous use of *prednisone* and cholestyramine, colestipol, barbiturates, rifampin, phenytoin, and theophylline, as these agents may decrease the action of prednisone. Decreased effects of anticoagulants, anticonvulsants, oral hypoglycemics and insulin, ambenonium, neostigmine, isoniazid, vaccines, anticholinesterases, salicylates, and somatrem may be caused by prednisone. Increased prednisone side effects may occur with the concurrent use of alcohol, salicylates, indomethacin, amphotericin B, digoxin, cyclosporine, and diuretics. Those agents that increase the action of prednisone include salicylates, estrogens, indomethacin, oral contraceptives, ketoconazole, and macrolide antibiotics. Potassium deficiency may result with the simultaneous use of aloe, buckthorn, rhubarb, and senna. The most common adverse effects of *prazosin HcL* include marked hypotension (with the first dose, which is the reason for the gradual increase in dosing), dizziness, drowsiness, headache, fatigue, paresthesias, depression, palpitations, syncope, tachycardia, nausea and vomiting, edema, and dyspnea. With *prazosin HcL* drug-to-drug interactions can occur with simultaneous use of antihypertensive agents, diuretics, beta-adrenergic blocking agents, and nifedipine, which will increase the antihypertensive effects of prazosin HcL. Severe postural hypotension can result with the concurrent use of propranolol and verapamil. Clonidine may decrease the antihypertensive effects of prazosin. No clinically significant drug-to-food/herbal interactions have been established. The most common adverse reactions of *pentoxifylline* are epistaxis, leukopenia, headache, tremors, dizziness, dyspepsia, nausea, vomiting. Drug-to-drug interactions may occur with the simultaneous use of *pentoxifylline* and ciprofloxacin and cimetidine, which may increase levels of toxicity. Additive hypotension may occur with antihypertensives and nitrates. The simultaneous use with warfarin, heparin, aspirin, nonsteroidal anti-inflammatory agents (NSAIDs), cefoperazone, cefotetan, plicamycin, valproic acid, clopidogrel, ticlopidine, eptifibatide, tirofiban, or thrombolytic agents may increase the risk of bleeding. Drug-to-food interactions are not established. Drug-to-herbal interactions are seen with the concurrent use of anise, arnica, asafetida, chamomile, clove, dong quai, fenugreek, feverfew, garlic, ginger, gingko biloba, grapeseed extract, evening primrose oil, Panax ginseng, and licorice resulting in increased bleeding potential, tolbutamide, tamoxifen, torsemide, fluvastatin, and warfarin.

7. Discuss medical and nursing management of complications of Buerger's disease. Ulceration and gangrene are common complications of Buerger's disease. They may occur early in the course of the disease, with gangrene usually occurring in one extremity at a time. The history of the condition is important in determining venous or arterial cause. Cultures of the ulcer(s) are necessary to determine whether the infecting agent is the primary cause of the ulcer(s). After the circulatory status has been assessed and determined to be adequate for healing, surgical dressings can be used to promote a moist environment. If the ulcer(s) is infected, oral antibiotics are prescribed, because topical antibiotics have not proven to be effective with leg ulcers. To promote wound healing, the wound is kept clean of drainage and necrotic tissue. Wound dressings vary, with the simplest method being the use of a wound contact material (e.g., Tegapore) next to the wound bed and cover it with gauze. However, deep wounds and infected wounds are more appropriately treated with other dressings.

8. **Discuss surgical management of complications of Buerger's disease.** If gangrene of a toe develops as a result of arterial occlusive disease in the leg, a below-the-knee amputation or an above-the-knee amputation is necessary. Indications for amputation include worsening gangrene, severe rest pain, or fulminating sepsis. If the wound is not infected, a traditional amputation (closed or flap) is performed. If the wound is infected, a guillotine (open) amputation is done. In this type of amputation, the surgeon does not close the stump with a skin flap immediately but leaves it open, allowing the wound to drain freely. The infected wound is treated with antibiotics and bed rest. Once the infection is completely eradicated, the client undergoes another surgery for stump closure.

9. **Discuss Buerger-Allen exercise.** Ask the client to lie flat, then elevate the legs above the heart for two minutes or until blanching of the skin occurs. Instruct the client to allow the legs to be dependent; exercise the feet approximately three minutes or until the legs are pink. Instruct the client to lie flat for approximately five minutes, then repeat the entire procedure three times each day. These instructions should be written out, and it should be emphasized to the client that prolonged and severe pain during exercise is contraindicated and must be reported to the primary health care provider.

10. **Discuss client education for Buerger's disease.** The client must avoid constricting clothes. The client should comply with discharge instructions. The client must stop smoking and dress appropriately in cold temperature. The client should report to the health care provider intolerable pain and discomfort in the extremities, since this type of pain may be an indicator of occlusion of a vessel, requiring emergency surgery such as a thrombectomy.

References

Broyles, B. E. (2005). *Medical-Surgical Nursing Clinical Companion*. Durham, NC: Carolina Academic Press.

"Buerger's Disease (Thromboangiitis Obliterans)." (August 2004). Available at www.emedicine.com

Corbet, J. V. (2004). *Laboratory Tests and Diagnostic Procedures with Nursing Diagnoses* (6th ed.). Upper Saddle River, NJ: Prentice Hall.

Gahart, B. L. and Nazareno, A. R. (2005). *2005 Intravenous Medications*. St. Louis: Elsevier Mosby.

Heitz, U. and Horne, M. M. (2005). *Mosby's Pocket Guide Series: Fluid, Electrolyte, and Acid-Base Balance*. St. Louis: Mosby.

Huether, S. E. and McCance, K. L. (2004). *Understanding Pathophysiology* (3rd ed.). St. Louis: Mosby.

Ignatavicius, D. D. and Workman, M. L. (2006). *Medical-Surgical Nursing across the Health Care Continuum* (5th ed.). Philadelphia: W. B. Saunders.

Spratto, G. R. and Woods, A. L. (2005). *2005 Edition: PDR Nurse's Drug Handbook*. Clifton Park, NY: Thomson Delmar Learning.

CASE STUDY 2

Primary Raynaud's Disease/ Raynaud's Phenomenon

GENDER

F

AGE

45

SETTING

- Health care provider's office

ETHNICITY/CULTURE

- White American

PREEXISTING CONDITIONS

- Carpal tunnel syndrome

COEXISTING CONDITIONS

- Paternal grandmother and mother have Raynaud's disease

LIFESTYLE

- Works as an executive secretary in a law firm
- Plays the piano for Sunday school
- Drinks at least six cups of coffee daily for several years

COMMUNICATION

DISABILITY

- Intermittent pain in the hands

SOCIOECONOMIC STATUS

- Low

SPIRITUAL/RELIGIOUS

- Presbyterian

PHARMACOLOGIC

- Enteric-coated aspirin (acetylsalicylic acid)
- Nifedipine (Procardia)

PSYCHOSOCIAL

- Anxiety

LEGAL

ETHICAL

ALTERNATIVE THERAPY

- Stress management
- Immersing hands in warm water

PRIORITIZATION

- Control pain

DELEGATION

- RN
- Client education

THE RESPIRATORY AND IMMUNE SYSTEMS

Level of difficulty: Easy

Overview: This case involves a thorough assessment of the client's complaints and provides prescribed medications and alternative therapy to reduce causative factors.

Client Profile

Ms. E is a 45-year-old executive secretary who is seen in her primary health care provider's office with complaints of attacks of pallor of the digits of both hands. On further discussion with the health care provider, Ms. E reports that six months ago she noticed a pattern of the digits whereby the digits are pale then a bluish-purple discoloration, with feelings of cold, tingling, and discomfort of the fingers. However, she reports that the symptoms have become worse, causing her to seek medical advice. Her vital signs on arrival to the office are:

Blood pressure: 110/74
Pulse: 74
Respirations: 14
Temperature: 98.6° F

She is 5′4″ and weighs 140 pounds.

Case Study

Ms. E denies previous medical or surgical history upon initial interview. After the history and physical assessment are done, serum labs for antinuclear antibody test and erythrocyte sedimentation rate (ESR) are drawn and sent to the lab. Ms. E is instructed by the health care provider to return to the office in three days from today's date for results of these labs and confirmation of the disease pathology. The health care provider informs her to take two acetaminophen (Tylenol) tablets every six hours until she returns for a follow-up visit in three days. Ms. E returns to the office as scheduled and reports that the pain of the digits did recur but that she immersed her hands in warm water, practiced stress management, and used acetaminophen as suggested, all of which made the pain tolerable. The health care provider discussed the findings of the lab tests with her: the antinuclear antibody test is negative and ESR is normal; her digits are pale, and when palpated, she reports a feeling of numbness and pain. The diagnosis of Raynaud's disease, or Raynaud's phenomenon, is confirmed. Ms. E is given a follow-up appointment of three months.

Questions

1. Discuss the pathophysiology of Raynaud's disease.

2. What is the three-color presentation of Raynaud's disease?

3. Discuss the goal of clinical management for the client with Raynaud's disease.

4. Discuss the common nursing diagnoses and expected outcomes for the client with Raynaud's disease.

5. What are the purposes for the prescribed orders?

Questions (continued)

6. What are the most common adverse reactions, drug-to-drug, drug-to-food/herbal interactions for the prescribed medications?

7. Discuss other medications that could be prescribed for the treatment of Raynaud's disease.

8. Discuss the traditional treatment of choice for Raynaud's disease when drug therapy does not alleviate the severe symptoms.

9. Discuss alternative/complementary therapy that may be effectively used with Raynaud's disease.

10. Discuss client's education for Raynaud's disease.

Questions and Suggested Answers

1. **Discuss the pathophysiology of Raynaud's disease.** Raynaud's disease is an episodic vasospasm that produces closure of the small arteries in the distal extremities in response to cold, vibration, or emotional stimuli. When exposed to cold, the body naturally responds by trying to maintain its core temperature, in part through vasoconstriction of the distal peripheral arteries and arterioles. However, in Raynaud phenomenon, a vascular disorder triggered by cold or emotional stress, an exaggerated vasoconstriction and vasospasm of the digital arteries and arterioles occurs. The fingers, and less often, the toes are affected; earlobes, lips, nose, and nipples may also be affected. Episodes can last from minutes to hours, and severity can range from mild and annoying to severe and debilitating, depending on the extent of tissue ischemia and whether it progresses to necrosis.

2. **What is the three-color presentation of Raynaud's disease?** Initially, there is the development of pallor (white color) which is caused by intense vasoconstriction or spasm in the digital arteries. As the episode progresses, triphasic color changes from white (pallor) to blue (cyanosis) to red (rubor) are seen in the most severe cases, although typical color changes are biphasic: pallor followed by rubor. Eventually vasoconstriction causes pallor of one or more of the fingertips, after which reactive hyperemia instigates rubor. If vasoconstriction is prolonged (causing desaturation of blood in the capillaries), cyanosis can occur although usually only in more advanced cases.

3. **Discuss the goal of clinical management for the client with Raynaud's disease.** The goal of clinical management for Raynaud's disease is to decrease the number of vasospastic episodes with the implementation of nonpharmacologic and pharmacologic interventions. Pharmacologic management will achieve dilation of blood vessels, relaxing of arterial walls, and improvement of circulation, which will reduce the frequency and severity of attacks.

4. Discuss the common nursing diagnoses and expected outcomes for the client with Raynaud's disease.

Nursing diagnosis: Altered tissue perfusion R/T peripheral vasospasm

Expected outcome: The client will exhibit signs of improved tissue perfusion as seen with decreased frequency of vasospastic episodes and the ability to carry out activities of daily living with minimal discomfort or pain. There will be an absence of fingertip or nail bed ulcerations.

Nursing diagnosis: Body image disturbance R/T physical changes caused by the disease process

Expected outcome: The client should verbalize understanding of changes in body image and freely discuss feelings with health care professionals and significant others, and demonstrate appropriate problem-solving techniques for coping with body changes.

Nursing diagnosis: Deficient knowledge R/T condition, treatment, and health maintenance

Expected outcome: The client will verbalize critical factors that cause and aggravate the disease (e.g., cigarette smoking, cold weather, stress) and state that prevention of recurrent episodes are possible with compliance of treatment regimen and follow-up care.

The following are prescribed:

- Enteric-coated aspirin (acetylsalicylic acid) 650 mg PO two times per day
- Nifedipine (Procardia) 10 mg PO three times per day

5. What are the purposes for the prescribed orders? *Aspirin* is an antiplatelet agent that powerfully inhibits platelet aggregation, improving blood flow and normal tissue perfusion. It is beneficial for this client because it is the altered tissue perfusion that is a major cause of the pain and discomfort the client experiences. *Nifedipine* is a calcium channel-blocking agent with a strong vasodilating effect that relaxes smooth muscles of the arterioles. It does this by blocking the influx of calcium into the cells, which reduces the number of vasospastic attacks.

6. What are the most common adverse reactions, drug-to-drug, drug-to-food/herbal interactions of the prescribed medications? The most common adverse reactions of aspirin are nausea, heartburn, and stomach pains. Enteric coated aspirin reduces the gastrointestinal intestinal (GI) effects, but they may still occur after the drug is broken down in the GI system. Drug-to-drug interactions of aspirin include the simultaneous use of aminosalicylic acid, which may increase the risk of salicylate toxicity. With the use of methotrexate, toxicity is increased, and low doses of salicylates may antagonize uricosuric effects of probenicid and sulfinpyrazone. Herbal interactions may occur with the simultaneous use of feverfew, garlic, ginger, and gingko, which may increase the risk of bleeding. The most common adverse reactions of *nifedipine* are dizziness, lightheadedness, headache, facial flushing, heat sensation, peripheral edema, and diarrhea. With *nifedipine* drug-to-drug interactions may occur with the simultaneous use of fentanyl, antihypertensives, nitrates, alcohol or quinidine, which may cause additive hypotension. The concurrent use with digoxin may increase serum digoxin levels and toxicity. Concurrent use with beta-blockers, disopyramide, or phenytoin may result in bradycardia, conduction defects, or CHF. The concurrent use with cimetidine, diltiazem, itraconazole, quinupristin/dalfopristin, ranitidine, rifampin, and propranolol may decrease the metabolism and increase risk for nifedipine toxicity. Use with barbiturates decreases nifedipine's effects and used with warfarin, cyclopsporine, magnesium sulfate, tacolimus, theophylline, and vincristine increases the effects of these agents. Grapefruit juice increases serum levels and effect, and St. John's Wort increases the metabolism of nifedipine, thus decreasing its serum levels. With the simultaneous use of melatonin an increase blood pressure and heart rate may occur.

7. **Discuss other medications that could be prescribed for the treatment of Raynaud's disease.** Currently, calcium-channel blockers (CCB) are the first-line drug therapy for Raynaud's disease. Diltiazem (Cardizem) is a CCB that also relaxes the smooth muscle of the arterioles, and enhance blood flow, decreasing vasospastic attacks. Another medication that may be prescribed are sympatholytic agents (e.g., a-adrenergic-receptor blockers): phenoxybenzamine (Dibenzyline), an alpha-blocker which has been found useful in treating vascular disorders such as Raynaud's. It is effective in Raynaud's disease because it directly blocks the alpha-adrenergic receptors and is therefore very useful in the treatment of vasospastic disorders. Drugs currently being researched to treat Raynaud's disease include angiotensin II-receptor blockers such as losartan potassium, that works to selectively blocks the binding of angiotensin II, and cause vasodilation of arteries and aterioles, with improvement of blood flow. Cilostazol (Petal) is a platelet inhibitor that suppresses platelet aggregation, and in doing so, promotes vasodilation, and decrease pain related to altered tissue perfusion. Sympatholytic agents such as prazosin (Minipress) and doxazosin (Cardura) have been used to manage Raynaud's disease. They are effective because they counteract the actions of norepinephrine, a catecholamine that is a strong vasoconstrictor, and in doing so, promote blood flow and decrease frequency of attacks.

8. **Discuss the traditional treatment of choice for Raynaud's disease when drug therapy does not alleviate the severe symptoms.** When drug therapy

does not alleviate the severe symptoms of Raynaud's disease, a surgical procedure may be performed. If the upper extremity digits are involved, the health care provider does a sympathetic ganglionectomy. If the severity of symptoms is in the lower extremity digits, the lumbar sympathectomy, whereby the sympathetic nerve fibers that cause vasoconstriction of blood vessels are cut.

9. Discuss alternative/complementary therapy that may be effectively used with Raynaud's disease. Biofeedback workshops are alternative type of strategies that have been beneficial for clients with Raynaud's disease. It is beneficial because it relieves stress, which is a factor in the development of symptoms seen in Raynaud's disease.

10. Discuss client's education for Raynaud's disease. Do not discontinue nifedipine without medical instructions. Sudden withdrawal of nifidepine may cause severe hypertension and other adverse reactions. Do not use grapefruit juice while taking nifedipine. Grapefruit juice will increase the serum levels of nifidepine and risk for toxicity. Take action during an attack, such as warming the hands or feet when cold. Take time to relax, or get out of a stressful situation, then practice relaxation technique. If you are trained in biofeedback use it along with warming the hands or feet in water to help lessen the attack. Exercise regularly after getting clearance from your primary health care provider. Exercise promotes an overall well-being, increases energy level, helps control weight, and promotes restful sleep, which will decrease the attacks. Emphasis should be placed on the importance of follow-up care since persons with Raynaud's disease may experience bouts of exacerbation, and will need modification of current medication regimen.

References

Black, J. M. and Hawks, J. H. (2005). *Medical-Surgical Nursing: Clinical Management for Positive Outcomes*. Philadelphia: W. B. Saunders.

Broyles, B. E. (2005). *Medical-Surgical Nursing Clinical Companion*. Durham, NC: Carolina Academic Press.

Corbet, J. V. (2004). *Laboratory Tests and Diagnostic Procedures with Nursing Diagnoses* (6th ed.). Upper Saddle River, NJ: Prentice Hall.

Gahart, B. L. and Nazareno, A. R. (2005). *2005 Intravenous Medications*. St. Louis: Mosby.

Huether, S. E. and McCance, K. L. (2004). *Understanding Pathophysiology* (3rd ed.). St. Louis: Mosby.

Ignatavicius, D. D. and Workman, M. L. (2006). *Medical-Surgical Nursing across the Health Care Continuum* (5th ed.). Philadelphia: W. B. Saunders.

Reilly, A. and Snyder, B. (2005). "Raynaud Phenomenon." *American Journal of Nursing* 105(8): 57–65.

Skidmore-Roth, L. (2006). *Mosby's Handbook of Herbs & Natural Supplements* (3rd ed.). St. Louis: Mosby.

Spratto, G. R. and Woods, A. L. (2005). *2005 Edition: PDR Nurse's Drug Handbook*. Clifton Park, NY: Thomson Delmar Learning.

CASE STUDY 3

Cerebral Vascular Accident

GENDER

M

AGE

48

SETTING

- Home

ETHNICITY/CULTURE

- Black American

PREEXISTING CONDITION

- Carotid stenosis/hyperlipidemia

COEXISTING CONDITION

- Diabetes
- Hypertension
- Family history

LIFESTYLE

- Bank manager, works 5 days per week

COMMUNICATION

DISABILITY

- Left-sided weakness

SOCIO-ECONOMIC STATUS

- Middle

SPIRITUAL/RELIGIOUS

- Methodist

PHARMACOLOGIC

- Heparin sodium IV
- Aspirin (acetylsalicylic acid)
- Labetalol HcL (Normodyne)
- Felodipine (Plendil)

PSYCHOSOCIAL

- Anxiety
- Depression
- Emotional liability

LEGAL

ETHICAL

- Is the client entitled to disability benefits due to the left-sided weakness?

ALTERNATIVE THERAPY

- Traditional healers/modern medicine

PRIORITIZATION

- Safety
- Reduce blood pressure
- Medication administration
- Prevent complications

DELEGATION

- RN skilled in neurological assessment
- Documentation

M
O
D
E
R
A
T
E

THE CARDIOVASCULAR AND LYMPHATIC SYSTEMS

Level of difficulty: Moderate

Overview: This multifaceted case involves a thorough assessment of past medical history such as transient ischemic attacks, coronary artery disease, or long history of alcohol intake. The nurse must use critical thinking skills to provide effective care to a client with partial speech deficit.

Client Profile

Mr. R is a 48-year-old male who lives at home with his older sister. Five months ago he was discharged from the hospital with a diagnosis of unstable angina. He is 5′6″ and weighs 240 pounds.

Case Study

Mr. R is brought to the hospital emergency department (ED) from his primary health care provider's office via emergency medical services (EMS). On arrival to the ED, Mr. R complains of occasional chest pain that goes away whenever he uses sublingual nitroglycerin (NTG). He also complains of dizziness, especially when moving from a lying to sitting or standing position. His sister had accompanied him to the primary health care provider for routine follow-up care and is present in the ED during this interview. His sister reports that Mr. R has weakness in the lower extremities and infrequent headaches that are transient in nature. She informs the triage nurse that whenever he complains of "these headaches," she uses an electronic blood pressure machine to monitor his blood pressure, which is infrequently elevated. His vital signs on admission are:

Blood pressure: 210/160
Pulse: 84
Respirations: 20
Temperature: 99.6°F

Records from his primary health care provider's office document complaints of occasional chest pains that are relieved by NTG. Although he has minimal left-sided weakness related to a mild stroke six months ago, his sister informs the triage nurse that he is able to stand for appropriate periods of time with the use of a cane but needs assistance to get out of bed. A recent Doppler study of the lower extremities done at the health care provider's office is negative, but a Technetium-99m sestamibi scan (a test that provides higher-quality images of the coronary arteries and perfusion images) shows mild decreased perfusion of the anterior wall with a left ventricular ejection fraction of 36%. A duplex Doppler ultrasound scanning finds a 90% stenosis of the right carotid. His past medical history (PMH) reveals: peripheral vascular disease (PVD), unstable angina pectoris, coronary artery disease (atherosclerosis), diabetes mellitus type II (NIDDM), hypertension (HTN), a right cerebral vascular accident (CVA) seven years ago, and a mild stroke six months ago. His medical records from the health care provider's office show that he has prescriptions for simvastatin (Zocor) 20 mg PO daily, aspirin (acetylsalicylic acid) 325 mg PO daily, clonidine (Catapress) 0.2 mg PO daily, glizipide (Glucotrol) 5 mg PO daily, and docusate sodium (Colace) 100 mg PO three times per day. His social history reveals years of cigarette smoking and occasional alcohol intake. Past surgical history (PSH) indicates: triple vessel coronary artery bypass graft (CABG) six years ago and a left carotid endarterectomy two years ago. Mr. R is transferred from the ED to the medical intensive care unit (MICU) and placed on telemetry. On physical assessment, bruits are heard over both right and left carotids. Admission labs:

Glucose: 107 mg/dl
Blood urea nitrogen (BUN): 22 mg/dl
Creatinine: 1.2
Sodium (Na): 136
Potassium (K+): 4.8
Calcium: 8.3
High-density lipoprotein (HDL): 45
Low-density lipoprotein (LDL): 216
Very low density lipoprotein (VLDL): 75%
Creatine phosphokinase-myoglobin (CPK-MB): 2.54
Creatine phophokinase (CPK): 320
Prothrombin time (PT): 15.2 seconds, Control: 14.2 seconds
Partial thromboplastin time (PTT): 49.6 seconds, Control: 29.9 seconds
White blood cell (WBC) count: 14.4
Red blood cell (RBC) count: 3.37
Hemoglobin (Hgb): 11 g/dL
Hematocrit (Hct): 34.8%
Platelet count (PLT): 293
Urine for glucose, ketones, and culture and sensitivity: negative
Arterial blood gas (ABG):

pH: 7.38
PaO_2: 94
$PaCO_2$: 35
HCO_3: 24

An electrocardiogram (EKG) showed fine atrial fibrillation, chest X-ray with normal findings. During the night, Mr. R develops progressive left-sided weakness and expressive aphasia. A CT angiography finds vascular occlusion and decreased perfusion to areas of the brain. A diagnosis of cerebral vascular accident (CVA) with left-sided weakness related to thrombotic stroke is confirmed.

Questions

1. Discuss the pathophysiology of CVA.

2. Discuss different types of strokes.

3. Discuss verbal deficits that occur with CVA.

4. Discuss the relationship of hypertension and CVA.

5. Discuss clinical manifestations of CVA.

6. Discuss complications of CVA.

7. What alternative therapies may be used to control hypertension and prevent recurrence of CVA?

8. What are the purposes for the prescribed orders?

9. What are the most common adverse reactions, drug-to-drug, and drug-to-food/herbal interactions for the prescribed medications?

10. Discuss client education and home-care management for hypertension and CVA.

Questions and Suggested Answers

1. Discuss the pathophysiology of CVA. CVA occurs when there is a sudden loss of brain function resulting from disruption of the blood supply to a part of the brain. It is primarily a neurologic problem in the United States and in the world. Although there are various types of strokes, the result is an interruption in the blood supply to the brain causing temporary or permanent loss of movement, thought, memory, speech, or sensation.

2. Discuss different types of strokes. *Ischemic strokes* are subdivided into three different types: large artery thrombosis, small penetrating artery thrombosis, and cardiogenic embolic stroke. Large artery thrombotic strokes are due to atherosclerosis of the large blood vessels within the brain. Thrombus formation may also occur, and along with the atherosclerosis, there is a decrease in blood supply to the brain, resulting in ischemia and infarction. Small penetrating artery thrombotic strokes affect one or more vessels and are the most common type of ischemic stroke. Small artery thrombotic strokes are also called lacunar strokes because of the cavity that is created once the infarcted brain tissue dissipates. Cardiogenic embolic strokes are associated with cardiac arrhythmias, usually atrial fibrillation. In this type of stroke, emboli originate from the heart and circulate to the cerebrovasculature, resulting in a stroke (most commonly in the left middle cerebral artery). Embolic strokes may be prevented with the use of anticoagulation in clients with atrial fibrillation. *Hemorrhagic strokes* are the result of bleeding into the brain tissue or into a space such as the subarachnoid space. Hemorrhagic strokes can be caused by arteriovenous malformations, aneurysm rupture, certain drugs (anticoagulants and amphetamines), or uncontrolled hypertension. Because illicit drugs can cause hemorrhagic strokes, some clinicians may obtain a toxicology screen for drugs if the client is younger than 40 years of age. Extradural hemorrhage (epidural hemorrhage) is a neurosurgical emergency and requires urgent care if the client is to survive. It usually follows skull fracture with a tear of the middle artery or other meningeal artery. Subdural hemorrhage (excluding acute subdural hemorrhage) is basically the same as an epidural hemorrhage, except that in subdural hematoma usually a bridging vein is torn. Subarachnoid hemorrhage may occur as a result of trauma or hypertension, but the most common cause is a leaking aneurysm in the area of the circle of Willis and congenital arteriovenous malformations of the brain. Intracerebral hemorrhage is bleeding into the brain substance and is most common in clients with hypertension and cerebral atherosclerosis because degenerative changes from these diseases cause rupture of the vessel.

3. Discuss verbal deficits that occur with CVA. *Expressive aphasia* is a deficit in the ability to communicate and may involve any or all aspects of communication, including speaking, reading, writing, and understanding. However, most aphasias are partial rather than complete. Expressive aphasia occurs when the normal function of the inferior-posterior frontal area of the brain is altered due to interference of blood flow to the anterior cerebral artery. Mr. R is experiencing partial aphasia. In *receptive aphasia*, the client is unable to comprehend the spoken word. A client may be able to say words that are not easily understood. *Global aphasia* is a combination of both receptive and expressive aphasia.

4. Discuss the relationship of hypertension and CVA. Mr. R has a history of hypertension for several years and has been on prescribed antihypertensive medications under medical supervision. Prolonged history of hypertension results from a sustained increase in peripheral vascular resistance or an increase in circulating blood volume. If the hypertension is chronic, the long-standing vasoconstriction damages the walls of systemic blood vessels, which increases the risk of thrombosis due to a reduction of the lumen of the arteries and reduction of blood flow, resulting in thrombus formation over a period of time. History of atherosclerosis, peripheral vascular disease, and diabetes mellitus increases the risk for CVA because all of these diseases impair blood flow to arteries and veins, and increase the risk of thrombus formation. If clot formation breaks off, the potential for stroke becomes greater because the client is now at risk for thrombotic and embolic stroke. Atherosclerosis over a prolonged period of time obstructs the vessels (carotids) supplying the brain with blood. Because any part of the body may become ischemic when its blood supply is compromised by atherosclerotic lesions, an individual may experience various ischemic complications, which will result in a stroke.

5. **Discuss clinical manifestations of CVA.** *CVA* causes a wide variety of neurologic deficits, depending on the location of the lesion, the size of the area of inadequate perfusion, and the amount of collateral blood flow. The client may have various signs and symptoms such as numbness or weakness of the face, arm, or leg, especially on one side of the body; confusion or change in mental status; trouble speaking or understanding speech; visual disturbances; difficulty walking; dizziness or loss of balance or coordination; and sudden headache.

6. **Discuss complications of CVA.** *Hemiplegia* or paralysis of one side of the body results from damage to the motor area of the cortex or the pyramidal tract fibers. However, muscles of the thorax and abdomen are usually not paralyzed because they are innervated from both cerebral hemispheres. *Homonymous hemianopia* is defective vision or visual loss in the same half of the visual field of each eye, so the client sees only one-half of normal vision. Depth perception and visual perception of horizontal and vertical planes may also be impaired. *Respiratory infection* may develop because of impaired consciousness, which deprives the client of the ability to ventilate or cough and deep-breathe normally, increasing the risk of bacterial pneumonia. The immunocompromised state of the client interferes with the cough and gag reflex, therefore the client is at risk for aspiration pneumonia.

7. **What alternative therapies may be used to control hypertension and prevent recurrence of CVA?** Alternative therapies to control hypertension include biofeedback and progressive muscle relaxation. Biofeedback is a technique of physiological self-control using instruments that measure bodily processes such as skin temperature, heart rate, muscle electrical activity, and sometimes brain waves. Progressive muscle relaxation is a process of alternately tensing and relaxing muscle groups to promote awareness of subtle degrees of tension. It reduces anxiety and allows clients to experience a heightened sense of comfort.

The following are prescribed:

- Heparin sodium infusion 40,000 units in 1000 mL 0.9% normal saline at 40 mL/hr/24 hours
- Labetalol HcL (Normodyne) 20 mg IV, titrate to stabilize blood pressure 130/80
- Aspirin (acetylsalicylic acid) EC 325 mg PO daily
- Simvastatin (Zocor) 20 mg PO at bedtime
- Glizipide (Glucotrol) 5 mg PO daily
- Divalproex (Depakote) 15 mg/kg/daily PO
- Colace (Docosate sodium) 100 mg PO three times per day
- Human Regular Insulin (Humulin R) coverage: 0–180 mg/dL = none; 181–220 mg/dL, give two units; 221–250 mg/dL, give four units;

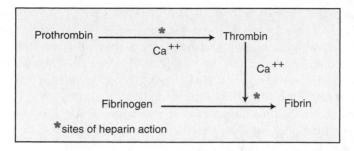

Final stages of the blood-clotting process; herapin exerts its anticoagulant activity by interfering with the conversion of prothrombin to thrombin.

251–300 mg/dL, give 6 units; 301–350 mg/dL, give eight units; above 350 mg/dL, give nine units and notify the health care provider
- IV 0.9% NaCL at 50 mL/hr
- Serum labs: glucose, WBC, CBC, PT, aPTT, CPK, LDL, creatinine daily

8. What are the purposes for the prescribed orders? *Heparin sodium IV* prevents clot formation by exerting direct effect on blood coagulation (clotting), and in doing so, enhances the inhibitory actions of anti-thrombin III (heparin cofactor) on the factors essential to normal blood clotting. When the actions of anti-thrombin are enhanced, the conversion of pro-thrombin to thrombin and fibrinogen to fibrin is suppressed, and forma-tion of clots is prevented. *Heparin* is given by constant infusion to maintain a consistent blood level. *Labetalol HcL* maintains optimum systolic blood pressure and maintains cerebral perfusion pressure. It is an autonomic nervous system agent with alpha/beta adrenergic properties that quickly lowers blood pressure by vasodilation and reduction of peripheral resis-tance. *Aspirin* inhibits platelet aggregation. It reduces the ability of clot for-mation, which helps to prevent the recurrence of a stroke. It is beneficial for this client, who has a positive history of cardiovascular problems, post-stroke, occluded carotid, and impaired peripheral vascular status. *Simvastatin*, an HMG CoA reductase inhibitor, for its effectiveness in low-ering low-density lipoprotein (LDL) cholesterol level, which is "bad" cho-lesterol, and increasing high-density-lipoprotein level, the "good" cholesterol, which would permit better blood flow, reducing the risk of a recurrent cerebral vascular accident. *Glipizide* stabilizes blood glucose lev-els. It stabilizes the blood glucose by directly stimulating functioning pan-creatic beta cells to secrete insulin. It also indirectly causes alteration in the numbers and sensitivity of peripheral insulin receptors, resulting in increased insulin binding, averting of elevated blood glucose levels. *Divalproex* decreases seizure activities by depressing abnormal neuron dis-charges in the central nervous system. *Colace* softens the stool and prevents straining at time of defecation. It softens the stool by pulling water into the colon, softens the stool, making it possible for the client to defecate without straining. Straining during defecation could result in increase in intracranial pressure and rupture of cerebral vessels. *Human Regular Insulin* lowers glucose and prevents elevated glucose from resulting in complications. Although Mr. R has Type II diabetes mellitus, he has many current stressors, including hospitalization, that may cause the release of glucogenic hormones into the bloodstream and the increase in glucose levels. *Insulin sliding scale* guides treatment of occurring hyperglycemia. If hyperglycemia is not effectively managed, the client could develop complications such as hyperglycemic-hyperosmolar nonketotic syndrome (HHNKS). The *intravenous infusion of 0.9% NaCL* helps to maintain the concentration and volume of extracellular fluid and to help with the regulation of acid-base balance. An *intravenous rate of 50 mL per hour* keeps the vein open and provides access for medication administration. Laboratory evaluation of the client with ischemic stroke is important in managing care. The *glucose* is monitored because hypoglycemia is a common electrolyte abnormality manifested by clients with ischemic stroke and is easily corrected. The *CBC* provides key information regarding hemoglobin and hematocrit deficiencies in oxygen-carrying capacity. It also provides information on the WBC count, which is high on admission and will need reevaluation. The presence of *prothrombin time (PT) and activated partial thromboplastin time (aPTT)* are needed to manage heparin and Coumadin, if prescribed. The CPK is very elevated on admission and needs continued evaluation to prevent complications. Elevated CPK may be a response to the CVA. The *LDL* is evaluated daily because it is high on admission. Daily evaluation will guide modification of Simvastatin therapy.

9. What are the most common adverse reactions, drug-to-drug, drug-to-food/herbal interactions of the prescribed medications? The most common adverse reactions of *heparin sodium* are anemia and transient thrombocytopenia. Drug-to-drug interactions may be seen with the simultaneous use of nonsteroidal anti-inflammatory agents (NSAIDs), aspirin, clopidogrel, dipyridamole, warfarin, thrombolytics, some penicillins, ticlopidine, abciximab, eptifibatide, tirofiban, quinidine, cefamandole, cefmetazole, cefoperazone, cefotetan, plicamycin, valproic acid, and dextran, which may increase the risk of bleeding. Nitroglycerin IV, digoxin, tetracyclines, nicotine, and antihistamines may decrease anticoagulant effects. Protamine sulfate may antagonize the effects of *heparin.* Drug-to-food/herbal interactions may occur with the simultaneous use of feverfew, gingko, ginger and valerian, arnica, anise, chamomile, clove, dong quai, and Panax ginseng, which could increase the risk of bleeding. The most common adverse reactions of *aspirin* are heartburn, dyspepsia, epigastric distress, stomach pains, and nausea. Drug-to-drug interactions may occur with the simultaneous use of

ammonium chloride, which may decrease renal elimination and increase toxicity; anticoagulants and thrombolytic agents, ticlopidine, clopidogrel, torfiban, and eptifibatide, which may increase the risk of bleeding; oral hypoglycemic agents, which may increase hypoglycemic activity; and corticosteroids, which may increase ulcerogenic effects and decrease serum salicylate levels. Drug-to-food/herbal interactions may occur with the simultaneous use of garlic, ginger, gingko, feverfew, anise, arnica, chamomile, clove, Panax ginseng, and licorice. The most common adverse reactions of *simvastatin* are insomnia, leukopenia, thrombocytopenia, hyperlipidemia, arthralgias, abdominal cramps, constipation, flatus, and tremor. Drug-to-drug interactions may occur with the simultaneous use of warfarin sodium, which may increase prothrombin time. Cyclosporine, ketoconazole, diltiazem, nicardipine, verapamil, clotrimazole, fluconazole, itracomazole, clarithromycin, erythromycin, troleandomycin, metoclopramide, cimetidine, danazol, and protease inhibitor antiretrovirals greatly increase blood levels. Rifampin increases metabolism significantly, decreasing blood levels. Carbamazepine, phenobarbital, phenytoin, rifabutin, and rifapentine decrease the blood level of *simvastatin.* Simultaneous use with liver-virus vaccine may decrease antibody response and increase risk for adverse reactions. The simultaneous use with protease inhibitors may increase *simvastatin's* serum levels and increase the risk for myopathy and rhabdomyolysis. Drug-to-food/herbal interactions may occur if grapefruit juice is a part of the diet if there is concomitant use with Echinacea, melatonin, and St. John's Wort, which will increase the risk of toxicity. The most common adverse reaction of *colace* is diarrhea. Abdominal cramps and diarrhea may be present but are minimal. There are no clinically significant drug-to-drug/food/herbal interactions established. The most common adverse reactions of *human regular insulin* are lipodystrophy, profuse sweating, hypoglycemia, nausea, tremulousness, and palpitations. Drug-to-drug interactions may occur with the simultaneous use of steroids, MAO inhibitors, epinephrine, beta-blockers, and furosemide, which may antagonize glycemic effects. Thiazide diuretics, corticosteroids, diltiazem, dobutamine, thyroid preparations, estrogens, nicotine, protease inhibitor antiretrovirals, and rifampin may increase insulin requirements. Anabolic steroids (testosterone), alcohol, clofibrate, guanethidine, MAO inhibitors, most NSAIDs, oral hypoglycemic agents, sulfinpyrazone, tetracyclines, phenylbutazone, and warfarin may decrease insulin requirements. Drug-to-food/herbal interactions may occur with the simultaneous use of garlic; glucosamine, which may worsen blood glucose control; fenugreek, chromium, ginseng, and coenzyme Q-10, which may produce additive hypoglycemic effects.

10. Discuss client education and home-care management for hypertension and CVA. Gradual weight reduction is necessary to decrease and normalize blood pressure. Decrease salt intake to help with normalizing blood pressure.

Read labels of foods carefully to detect high salt content. Celery, onion, and garlic contain much salt, so limit or decrease their use. Decreasing dietary fat and increasing polyunsaturated fat helps to decrease blood pressure and cholesterol level. Remove the skin from all poultry before cooking. Limit caffeine to a minimum of one cup of coffee per day, because prolonged use of caffeine causes vasoconstriction resulting in hypertension. Alcohol intake needs to be carefully assessed and limited as much as possible. Instruct the client on the use of biofeedback to help reduce blood pressure. Instruct the client or significant other (S/O) how to lock the wheelchair and to keep it placed beside the bed on the client's unaffected side. The client should use the unaffected arm and leg to move the affected arm and leg. As the client's legs drop over the edge of the bed, the client should swing his body up to a sitting position by using the unaffected arm and leg. The client should then reach across the wheelchair and grasps the far arm of the chair, then turn and seat himself. Stress the importance of adherence to prescribed medications and follow-up care.

References

Broyles, B. E. (2005). *Medical-Surgical Nursing Clinical Companion*. Durham, NC: Carolina Academic Press.

Corbet, J. V. (2004). *Laboratory Tests and Diagnostic Procedures with Nursing Diagnoses* (6th ed.). Upper Saddle River, NJ: Prentice Hall.

Gahart, B. L. and Nazareno, A. R. (2005). *2005 Intravenous Medications*. St. Louis: Mosby.

Heitz, U. and Horne, M. M. (2005). *Mosby's Pocket Guide Series: Fluid, Electrolyte and Acid-Base Balance* (5th ed.). St. Louis: Mosby.

Huether, S. E. and McCance, K. L. (2004). *Understanding Pathophysiology* (3rd ed.). St. Louis: Mosby.

Ignatavicius, D. D. and Workman, M. L. (2006). *Medical-Surgical Nursing: Critical Thinking for Collaborative Care* (5th ed.). Philadelphia: W. B. Saunders.

Spratto, G. R. and Woods, A. L. (2005). *2005 Edition: PDR Nurse's Drug Handbook*. Clifton Park, NY: Thomson Delmar Learning.

Myocardial Infarction

GENDER

M

AGE

60

SETTING

- Hospital ED

ETHNICITY/CULTURE

- White American

PREEXISTING CONDITIONS

- Coronary artery disease

COEXISTING CONDITIONS

LIFESTYLE

- Electrical engineer

COMMUNICATION

DISABILITY

SOCIOECONOMIC STATUS

- Middle

SPIRITUAL/RELIGIOUS

- Presbyterian

PHARMACOLOGIC

- Atropine sulfate (Atropine)
- Nitroglycerin sublingual (Nitrostat)
- Morphine sulfate (Duramorph)
- Dobutamine HcL (Dobutrex)
- Lidocaine HcL (Xylocaine)
- Heparin sodium (Hepalean)
- Docusate sodium (Colace)

PSYCHOSOCIAL

- Anxiety
- Fear

LEGAL

ETHICAL

ALTERNATE THERAPY

PRIORITIZATION

- Pain management
- Thrombolytics
- Continuous telemetry

DELEGATION

- RN
- Client education

MODERATE

THE CARDIOVASCULAR AND LYMPHATIC SYSTEMS

Level of difficulty: Moderate

Overview: This case requires clinical competence to prioritize, triage, and delegate effectively to avoid further complications and possible death. The case also involves the ability to administer potent medications safely. It also requires a nurse who is knowledgeable and skilled in detecting dysrhythmias and is able to perform resuscitation if needed. This case involves astute implementation of care and effective delegation in a busy emergency department.

Client Profile

Mr. L is a 60-year-old electrical engineer who is 5'9" and weighs 182 pounds. He is admitted to the hospital emergency department (ED) from a cardiologist's office due to complaints of midsternal chest pain that did not go away with nitroglycerin (NTG). An electrocardiogram (EKG) reading reveals ST segment elevation and occasional premature ventricular contractions (PVC).

Case Study

On transfer to the hospital, Mr. L is anxious and expresses fear related to the current pain and past medical problems. He states he was diagnosed a month ago with a myocardial infarction. Records from the cardiologist's office indicate "Non-ST segment elevation MI one month ago." Mr. L denies allergies to food or drugs. Vital signs on admission are:

Blood pressure: 180/90 initially, then 140/80 thirty minutes later
Pulse: 58
Respirations: 22
Temperature: 98.9° F

Mr. L is anxious and restless at the time of admission to the ED but denies chest pain upon arrival in the triage area. A history and physical is done. A chest X-ray reveals clear lung fields. Serum labs for Troponin, complete blood count (CBC), prothrombin time (PT) and partial thromboplastin time (PTT), creatinine kinase (CK-MB), sodium (Na), and potassium (K+) levels are drawn and sent to the lab stat. Laboratory report reveals:

Troponin T: 0.4 ng/ml
Troponin I: 0.05 ng/mL
Creatinine kinase (CK-MB): 180 U/L
Complete blood count (CBC):
    White blood cell (WBC): 16,000/mm^3
    Hematocrit (Hct): 40%
    Hemoglobin (Hgb): 17 g/dl
Prothrombin time (PT): 11 seconds
Partial thromboplastin time (PTT): 60 seconds
Sodium (Na): 135 mEq/L
Potassium (K+): 4.8 mEq/L
Platelet count: 160,000/mm^3

While the primary nurse is gathering data for the nursing history, Mr. L complains of pain at the center (substernal) chest that is crushing with pressure and heaviness, radiating to both shoulders and arms. The nurse administers NTG 1/150 grain sublingually, but the pain is not relieved. A stat EKG reveals sustained ST segment elevation. The health care provider is called, and Mr. L is given a stat dose of morphine sulfate 8 mg intravenously, but the pain is not relieved. A diagnosis of acute myocardial infarction (AMI) is made. The primary nurse initiates streptokinase via infusion, and Mr. L is transferred to the medical intensive coronary unit (MICU) and placed on telemetry.

Questions

1. What are the locations of the left ventricular wall where MI usually occurs?

2. What are the major coronary vessels and the structures they perfuse?

3. Discuss the complications that may occur if these major arteries are obstructed.

4. Discuss the nursing focus of older adults with silent MI.

5. What are common nursing diagnoses for clients with MI?

6. What are the clinical manifestations of MI?

7. Discuss why morphine sulfate IV was prescribed for Mr. L during the acute phase of his MI.

8. What are the purposes for the prescribed orders?

9. What are the most common adverse effects of the prescribed medications?

10. Discuss the drug-to drug and drug-to-food/herbals interactions of the prescribed medications.

Questions and Suggested Answers

1. **What are the locations of the left ventricular wall where MI usually occurs?** Locations in the left ventricular wall where MI usually occurs are the anterior, lateral, septal, inferior, or posterior areas. MI usually occurs in these areas when the function of the left and right coronary arteries are altered. The left coronary artery supplies mainly the anterior and left lateral portions of the left ventricle, whereas the right coronary artery supplies most of the right ventricle as well as posterior part of the left ventricle. When these arteries become impaired or dysfunctional, nutritive blood supply to the heart is stopped. Obstruction of blood flow through these vessels results in death of a portion of the myocardium of the heart.

2. **What are the major coronary vessels and the structures they perfuse?** The left anterior descending coronary artery perfuses most of the left ventricular muscle mass and septum. The left circumflex coronary artery perfuses the posterior wall of the left ventricle, the sino-atrial (SA) node, the atrioventricular (AV) node, and portions of the left ventricular muscle. The right coronary artery perfuses the right ventricle, inferior portion of the left ventricle, the SA node, and the AV node.

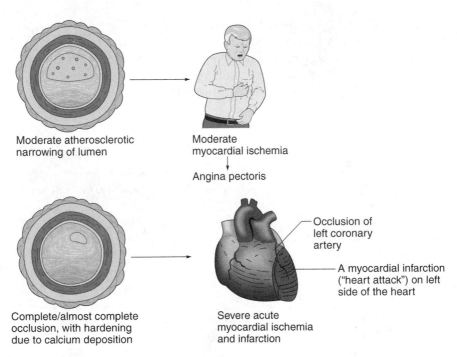

Moderate atherosclerotic narrowing of lumen

Moderate myocardial ischemia

Angina pectoris

Complete/almost complete occlusion, with hardening due to calcium deposition

Severe acute myocardial ischemia and infarction

Occlusion of left coronary artery

A myocardial infarction ("heart attack") on left side of the heart

Progressive atherosclerosis.

3. Discuss the complications that may occur if these major arteries are obstructed. Obstruction of the *left anterior descending* (LAD) artery causes anterior or septal MIs. Clients with anterior wall MIs are most likely to experience left ventricular heart failure and ventricular dysrhythmias because a large segment of the left ventricle may have been damaged. Obstruction of the *circumflex artery* may develop posterior wall MI or a lateral wall MI and sinus dysrhythmias. Obstruction of the right coronary artery results in inferior wall MIs, which causes significant damage to the right ventricle and would result in congested heart failure or pulmonary edema. Approximately 1.5 million people experience MIs annually in the United States and 200,000–300,000 die as a result.

4. Discuss the nursing focus of older adults with silent MI. Silent MI is recognized to affect 21–68% of older adults with coronary artery disease (CAD). The prevalence of clinically unrecognized MI diagnosed by routine EKGs in older persons varies from 21 to 68%. Most MIs in the older population do not present with clinical symptoms such as chest pain. Instead, clinicians will observe vague symptoms such as fatigue and nausea, with shortness of breath being the most pronounced. Some reasons for silent MI include the absence of chest pain in older adults due to reduction in their sensitivity to pain, because of nerve endings' response time.

5. **What are common nursing diagnoses for clients with MI?**

- Acute pain R/T biologic injury agents (imbalance between myocardial oxygen supply and demand)
- Ineffective cardiac tissue perfusion (cardiopulmonary) R/T interruption of arterial blood flow
- Decreased cardiac output R/T ineffective cardiac perfusion
- Activity intolerance R/T fatigue (caused by imbalance between oxygen supply and demand)
- Risk for injury R/T altered coagulation factors
- Ineffective coping R/T effects of acute illness and major changes in lifestyle
- Deficient knowledge R/T risk factors, condition, treatment, critical care environment, and lifestyle implications.

6. **What are the clinical manifestations of MI?** The key features of MI are substernal chest pressure radiating to the left arm, back, or jaw. The pain is relieved only with opioids and lasts for 30 minutes or more. Frequent symptoms are nausea, diaphoresis, dyspnea, feelings of fear and anxiety, dysrhythmias, fatigue, epigastric distress, and reports of feeling "short of breath."

7. **Discuss why morphine sulfate IV was prescribed for Mr. L during the acute phase of his MI.** Morphine sulfate is an opioid analgesic that is used to treat moderate to severe pain and is the drug of choice for the pain associated with MI. In addition, it relaxes cardiac muscle, improves cardiac perfusion, and relieves pulmonary congestion related to the acute pulmonary edema that accompanies left ventricular failure.

The following are prescribed:

- Atropine sulfate (Atropine) PRN stat for HR less than 60 beats per minute
- Nitroglycerin sublingual (Nitrostat) infusion 5 mcg/min in NS, titrate q3–5 min for desired response
- Morphine sulfate (Duramorph) 2–4 mg IV q1–2h PRN pain
- Diazepam (Valium) 5 mg PO q8h PRN anxiety
- Dobutamine (Dobutrex) 500 mg in 250 mL D5W at 5 mcg/kg/min for hypotensive episodes
- Lidocaine (Xylocaine) bolus (1 mg/kg) to be continued with lidocaine infusion
- Heparin sodium (Hepalean) 5,000 units in 0.9% NaCl 250 mL at 600 units (30 ml/hr)
- Docusate sodium (Colace) 100 mg PO three times per day
- Acetaminophen (Tylenol) 650 mg PO PRN temp greater than 101°

8. What are the purposes for the prescribed orders? *Acetaminophen* is a non-opiod analgesic and antipyretic agent that decreases temperature elevation and prevents an increase in metabolic rate to avoid additional stress on the body. *Acetaminophen* decreases fever by its direct affect on the hypothalamus heat-regulating center, resulting in peripheral vasodilation and heat loss. *Atropine sulfate* is an anticholinergic and antispasmodic agent used to increase the heart rate that is less than 60 to a normal of 60–100 beats per minute. Atropine HcL increases heart rate by blocking vagal impulses to the heart with resulting decrease in AV conduction time, increase in heart rate and cardiac output. *Nitroglycerin* (NTG) is a coronary vasodilator that is rapidly absorbed when administered sublingually. It relieves pain by enhancing blood flow to the coronary arteries. The anginal pain is secondary to decrease blood flow to the coronaries. If the pain is not relieved with this route of administration, intravenous NTG is administered to reduce myocardial workload and to relieve the pain. NTG also relieves anginal pain because it is a peripheral and arterial vasodilator that reduces afterload. It dilates coronary arteries and collateral channels in the heart and, in doing so, increases coronary blood flow. When coronary blood flow is increased, myocardial oxygen demand is decreased and there is increased oxygen available to the healthy tissue of the myocardium. *Morphine sulfate* is an opioid analgesic that relieves AMI pain. It relieves the pain by binding to the delta opioid receptors in the brain and spinal cord and activating the endogenous analgesia system through its potent analgesic effect. *Diazepam* is an anxiolytic used to relieve anxiety on a short-term basis. It acts by depressing activity in the brainstem and limbic system. When the brainstem is depressed, there is an increase of gamma-aminobutyric acid (GABA), an inhibitory neurotransmitter in the brain that functions to inhibit nerve transmission in the central nervous system (CNS). *Diazepam* also has specific receptor proteins, called receptor-binding sites, in the same areas of the brain that govern the release of GABA. It is the binding of diazepam with these receptor sites that produces anxiolytic effects including sedation and muscle relaxation. *Dobutamine* HcL is an inotropic cardiac stimulant that increases heart rate and cardiac output by stimulating the beta$_1$ receptors on the myocardium which increases contractility (positive inotropic) causing an increase stroke volume with resultant improvement in tissue perfusion to the damaged myocardium to prevent further injury. *Lidocaine HcL* is an antiarrhythmic agent used to prevent critical ventricular arrhythmias from progressing to MI or fatality. It prevents the progression of critical dysrhythmias by decreasing the sensitivity of the cardiac cell membrane to impulses and decreasing the cell's ability to depolarize on its own (decreasing automaticity, appropriately slowing ventricular rhythm). *Heparin* is a systemic anticoagulant that prevents thromboembolic complications from developing by exerting direct effect on blood

coagulation (clotting) by enhancing the inhibitory actions of antithrombin III and several factors essential to normal blood clotting. The result is the blocking of conversion of prothrombin to thrombin and fibrinogen to fibrin, preventing extension of existing thrombi and inhibiting formation of new clots. **Docusate sodium** is a stool softener that prevents constipation by its surface-active agent with emulsifying and wetting properties. The emulsifying effect lowers the surface tension of the intestines, permitting water and fats to penetrate and soften stools for easier passage. Mr. L will be on bed rest for an undetermined period of time. In addition, he will be receiving analgesics, which may alter peristalsis and enhance the risk for constipation. It is necessary that Mr. L avoid straining during defecation to prevent recurrence of an MI.

9. What are the most common adverse reactions of the prescribed medications? There are no clinically significant common adverse reactions of *acetaminophen* except hepatotoxicity, which may be seen in persons who are alcoholics or with overdoses. The most common adverse reactions of *atropine HcL* are dry mouth (xerostomia), blurred vision, and tachycardia. The most common adverse reactions of *NTG* are headache, dizziness, postural hypotension, and tachycardia. The most common adverse reactions of *morphine sulfate* are confusion, sedation, hypotension, pruritus, constipation, and nausea. The most common adverse reactions of *diazepam* are drowsiness, dizziness, and lethargy. The most common adverse reactions of *dobutamine HcL* are increased heart rate, increase blood pressure, and anginal pain. The most common adverse reactions of *lidocaine HcL* are confusion, apprehension, blurred vision, dizziness, nervousness, and drowsiness. Major adverse reactions include anaphylaxis, bradycardia, cardiac arrest, cardiovascular collapse, seizures, hypotension, respiratory depression, and cardiac arrythmias. The most common adverse reaction of *docusate sodium* is diarrhea that, in older clients, can lead to dehydration and electrolyte imbalances.

10. Discuss drug-to-drug and drug-to-food/herbal interactions of the prescribed medications. Drug-to-drug interactions may occur with the simultaneous use of *acetaminophen* and cholestyramine, which may decrease the absorption of acetaminophen, carbamazepine, phenytoin, and rifampin and may increase the potential for chronic hepatotoxicity. There are no clinically established drug-to-food/herbal interactions established. Drug-to-drug interactions with *atropine* may occur with the simultaneous use of amantadine, quinidine, and procainamide, which increases anticholinergic effects. There are no clinically significant drug-to-food/herbal interactions established. Drug-to-drug interactions may occur with *NTG* when used simultaneously with erectile dysfunction agents such as sildenafil, which can increase the risk of serious and potentially fatal hypotension. Additive hypotension may occur with the simultaneous use antihypertensives, acute ingestion of alcohol, beta blockers, calcium channel blockers, haloperidol, or phenothiazines. Agents having anticholinergic properties may decrease absorption of lingual, sublingual, or buccal nitroglycerin. There are no clinically significant drug-to-food/herbal interactions established. Drug-to-drug interactions occur with the simultaneous use of *morphine sulfate* and MAO inhibitors, which may result in unpredictable, severe reactions and hypertensive crisis. The simultaneous use of alcohol, sedative/hypnotics, clomipramine barbiturates, tricyclic antidepressants, and antihistamines increase CNS depression. Buprenorphine, nalbupine, butorphanol, or pentazocine may decrease analgesia. The simultaneous use with warfarin may increase the anticoagulant effect and concurrent use with cimetidine amitriptyline, clomipramine, and nortriptyline decreases the metabolism and may increase the effects of morphine. There are no clinically significant drug-to-food interactions established. Drug-to-herbal interactions may occur with the simultaneous use of kava-kava, valerian, and St. John's Wort, which may increase sedating effects. Drug-to-drug interactions may occur with *diazepam* when used simultaneously with CNS depressants, such as alcohol, and opioid analgesics, which may result in additive CNS depression. The simultaneous use of cimetidine with hormonal contraceptives, disulfiram, fluoxetine, isoniazid, ketoconazole, metoprolol, propoxyphene, propranolol, or valproic acid may decrease the metabolism of diazepam, enhancing its actions. If diazepam is used in conjunction with levodopa, it may decrease levodopa's effect, and its use with rifampin or barbiturates may increase the metabolism and decrease the effectiveness of diazepam. Drug-to-herb interactions may occur with the simultaneous use of kava-kava, valerian skullcap, chamomile, or hops, which can increase CNS depression. There are no clinically significant drug-to-food interactions established. Drug-to-drug interactions may occur with the simultaneous use of *dobutamine HcL* and cyclopropane and halothane, which may cause serious arrhythmias. Metoprolol and propranolol when used simultaneously with dobutamine HcL may prevent effective increase in cardiac output. There are no clinically significant drug-to-food/herbal interactions established. Drug-to-drug interactions may occur with the simultaneous use of *lidocaine HcL* with tocainide, which may cause cross-sensitivity and/or potentiate the actions of these agents. Quinidine increases the pharmacologic effects of lidocaine, and procainamide worsens neurologic and cardiac effects. There are no clinically significant drug-to-food/herbal interactions established. Drug-to-drug interaction may occur with the simultaneous use of *docusate sodium* and mineral oil, which may cause an increase in systemic absorption of mineral oil. Any food or herb taken to soften the stool or as a laxative will increase the effects of *docusate sodium* and will increase the risk of diarrhea. There are no clinically significant drug-to-food/herbal interactions established.

References

Broyles, B. E. (2005). *Medical-Surgical Nursing Clinical Companion*. Durham, NC: Carolina Academic Press.

Gahart, B. L. and Nazareno, A. R. (2005). *2005 Intravenous Medications*. St. Louis: Elsevier Mosby.

Huether, S. E. and McCance, K. L. (2004). *Understanding Pathophysiology* (3rd ed.). St. Louis: Mosby.

Ignatavicius, D. D. and Workman, M. L. (2006). *Medical-Surgical Nursing across the Health Care Continuum* (5th ed.). Philadelphia: W. B. Saunders.

Libster, M. (2002). *Delmar's Integrative Herb Guide for Nurses*. Albany, NY: Thomson Delmar Learning.

Lehne, R. A. (2003). *Pharmacology for Nursing Care* (5th ed.). Philadelphia: W. B. Saunders.

LeMone, P. and Burke, K. M. (2003). *Medical-Surgical Nursing: Critical Thinking in Client Care* (3rd ed.). Upper Saddle River, NJ: Prentice Hall.

Spratto, G. R. and Woods, A. L. (2005). *2005 Edition: PDR Nurse's Drug Handbook*. Clifton Park, NY: Thomson Delmar Learning.

Biventricular Heart Failure

GENDER

M

AGE

72

SETTING

- Hospital

ETHNICITY/CULTURE

- Black American

PREEXISTING CONDITIONS

COEXISTING CONDITIONS

- Coronary atherosclerosis
- Diabetes mellitus type 2
- Hypertension

LIFESTYLE

- Owner of several rental homes

COMMUNICATION

DISABILITY

SOCIOECONOMIC STATUS

- Middle

SPIRITUAL/RELIGIOUS

- Baptist

PHARMACOLOGIC

- Beta blockers
- Calcium-channel blockers
- Anti-lipid agents
- Oral hypoglycemic agents

PSYCHOSOCIAL

- Anxiety
- Depression

LEGAL

ETHICAL

ALTERNATIVE THERAPY

- Bittermelon, flaxseed, and ginseng

PRIORITIZATION

DELEGATION

- RN
- Client education

M O D E R A T E

THE CARDIOVASCULAR AND LYMPHATIC SYSTEMS

Level of difficulty: Moderate

Overview: This case study involves providing immediate care to the client using critical thinking skills to provide an initial assessment of the client so that delegation of the appropriate person can be correctly assigned, and emergency interventions be implemented. It also involves a systematic method of triaging the client safely for diagnostic studies that are necessary for accurate diagnosis. The case also involves maintaining effective communication with all healthcare personnel involved in emergency situations.

Client Profile

Mr. J is a 72-year-old male. He is 5'7" and weighs 188 pounds. He is found in the front of his home seated in a chair, holding his chest, and calling for help. Neighbors came to Mr. J's assistance and called emergency medical services (EMS). He was having difficulty breathing, so he was placed in an upright position in the chair and encouraged to relax. His family members were notified while the neighbors waited for the arrival of EMS. Mr. J was recently divorced after a marriage of 36 years. He has two sons and two daughters. The children are married, and his ex-wife lives in the same community where Mr. J presently resides.

Case Study

Mr. J is taken to the emergency department (ED) via EMS, is seen by the health care provider in the ED, and, after a quick assessment by the health care provider and triage nurse, is admitted to the intensive care unit (ICU). Mr. J's past medical history includes a long history of cigarette smoking, diabetes mellitus type 2, hyperlipidemia, hypertension, and stable angina pectoris. He reports being sedentary since his retirement five years ago and says his social activities at present include attending parties and gardening. Vital signs on admission are:

> Blood pressure: 170/100
> Pulse: 120
> Respirations: 24
> Temperature: 100.2° F

Also, there is 2+ pitting pedal edema. He is short of breath and orthopneic. He complains of being easily fatigued with minimal exercise, occasionally experiencing weakness, and frequently waking during the night to void. He also states that, at times, he awakes at night because he is acutely short of breath. On assessment, Mr. J has S_3 and S_4 gallop sounds, palpitations, and liver enlargement. He is placed on bed rest, continuous telemetry and two liters of oxygen via nasal cannula, and must be weighed daily. A chest X-ray is ordered and reveals pulmonary vascular congestion. An echocardiogram with Doppler-flow study finds decreased ejection fraction and ventricular hypertrophy, and a multigated angiographic (MUGA) scan confirms a decreased left ejection fraction as well as a decreased speed of contraction. A single-photon emission computed tomgraphy (SPECT) is done after Mr. J was more stabilized and reveals areas of decreased myocardial perfusion. An informed consent is signed by Mr. J for insertion of a central venous pressure (CVP) catheter. CVP readings with a pressure monitor register 14 mm Hg. Current medications brought by the family to the hospital are digoxin (Lanoxin), captopril (Capoten), furosemide (Lasix), spironolactone

(Aldactone), atenolol (Tenormin) and diltiazem (Cardizem), nicotinic acid (Niacin), rosiglitazone (Avandia), and docusate sodium (Colace). His significant other (SO) reports that Mr. J also uses herbal supplements (bittermelon, flaxseed, and ginseng). On auscultation, there are crackles (rales) over the lung fields bilaterally. Lab values are:

White blood cell (WBC) count: 9,000/mm^3
Hematocrit (Hct): 32.4%
Hemoglobin (Hgb): 14 g/dL
Sodium (Na): 130 mEq/L
Potassium (K+): 3 mEq/L
Chloride (Cl−): 99 mEq/L
Glucose: 130 mg/dL
Fingerstick glucose: 132
Blood urea nitrogen (BUN): 21 mg/dL
Creatinine: 1.4 mg/dL
Serum glutamic-oxaloacetic transaminase (SGOT): 44U/L
Serum glutamic-pyruvic transaminase (SGPT): 3.6 U/L
Protein total: 6 mg/dL
Total bilirubin: 1.8 mg/dL
Partial thromboplastin time (PTT): 38 seconds
Platelet count (PLT): 4,380,000/mm^3
High-density lipoprotein (HDL): 40 mg/dL
Low-density lipoprotein (LDL): 224 mg/dL
Triglycerides: 168 mg/dL
Ejection fraction: 35%

The multidisciplinary team reviewed the diagnostic reports and medications brought to the hospital by the client. A medical diagnosis of biventricular heart failure is confirmed. A registered dietitian reviews with Mr. J the nutritional plan of care that will be prescribed during hospitalization, a two-gram sodium diet.

Questions

1. What are some considerations for older adults with heart failure?

2. Which of the medications brought to the hospital by Mr. J has the risk of causing heart failure?

3. What are key manifestations of biventricular failure?

4. What are common nursing diagnoses for clients with heart failure?

5. What is the relationship between hypertension and the development of heart failure?

6. Discuss central venous pressure (CVP) catheter and significance of findings.

Questions (continued)

7. What complication could develop because of Mr. J's presenting symptoms on admission?

8. What are the purposes for the prescribed orders?

9. What are the most common adverse reactions for the prescribed medications?

10. Discuss the drug-to-drug, drug-to-food/herbal interactions of the prescribed medications.

11. Discuss specific nursing focus for the older client with heart failure.

12. What are the major areas of home care nurse assessment that are reimbursable by Medicare and other third-party payers?

13. Discuss client education and discharge planning for Mr. J.

Questions and Suggested Answers

1.   **What are some considerations for older adults with heart failure?** Older clients receiving loop diuretics such as furosemide are particularly prone to dehydration, especially if they have type 2 diabetes mellitus. They also are more likely to develop hypokalemia, likely in the case of Mr. J given that he is not receiving a potassium supplement. Hypokalemia increases the risk of digoxin toxicity, which is higher in the older client anyway due to decreased renal function (compounded by diabetes) for digoxin clearance. The dose of digoxin prescribed for Mr. J is at the high end of the normal range, making him more likely to develop toxicity than if he were receiving a lower dose. The nurse should check for orthostatic blood pressures in the client receiving loop diuretics to detect volume depletion. In light of the fact that Mr. J. also is receiving antihypertensive agents, the risk of hypotension is even greater. The client should be weighed daily to detect the development of a slow, progressive weight loss despite an adequate diet. The nurse also should observe for neck vein distention when the client is supine and for a loss of skin turgor, which may indicate dehydration.

2.   **Which of the medications brought to the hospital by Mr. J has the risk of causing heart failure?** The medication brought to the hospital with Mr. J that has the potential for causing heart failure is rosiglitazone maleate (Avandia). The drug is identified as having the potential for causing heart failure because one of its adverse effects is fluid retention.

3.   **What are key manifestations of biventricular failure?** Cough is an early manifestation of left-sided heart failure. Dyspnea and orthopnea are other common features that usually occur as a result of ineffective filling of the left side of the heart with blood returning from the lungs. As a result, fluid accumulates in the lungs causing a decrease in alveolar gas exchange.

Hypotension results from a decreased cardiac output; tachypnea occurs as the lungs attempt to compensate for the decrease in cardiac output; moist breath sounds are apparent due to the fluid accumulation in the lungs; fatigue results from inadequate cardiac output to meet the metabolic needs of body tissues. As a result of lung congestion, the client has an elevated pulmonary capillary wedge pressure and S_3 and S_4 gallops. As cardiac output decreases, manifestations of decreased perfusion in the brain are evident such as confusion, irritability, and restlessness.

Key manifestations of right-sided heart failure include peripheral edema resulting from fluid backing up in the periphery because the right side of the heart is unable to accommodate the normal venous return. This pitting edema is first apparent in the lower extremities but quickly also affects the upper extremities and into the neck veins. The liver becomes engorged with fluid, causing gastrointestinal symptoms such as nausea and anorexia.

4. What are common nursing diagnoses for clients with heart failure?

- Impaired gas exchange R/T pulmonary congestions and fluid volume excess
- Decreased cardiac output R/T altered contractility, preload, and afterload
- Activity intolerance R/T an imbalance between oxygen supply and demand
- Risk for impaired spontaneous ventilation R/T pulmonary congestion
- Deficient knowledge R/T condition, treatment, and home care

5. What is the relationship between hypertension and the development of heart failure? A client with a prolonged history of hypertension (HTN) has a high risk for heart failure over an extended period of time. Heart failure develops because in HTN there is vasoconstriction, which, if not corrected, will lead to increased peripheral resistance. If peripheral resistance is left untreated or clients are noncompliant with medication regimen for HTN, there is increased workload of the heart combined with diminished blood flow through the coronary arteries. The long-term effects are left ventricular hypertrophy, myocardial ischemia, and left heart failure. If the left ventricle fails, the right ventricle will be affected and eventually the client would develop biventricular failure. Regardless which side of the heart hypertrophies first, the other side will eventually be effected due to incomplete emptying of the cardiac chambers and decreased cardiac output.

6. Discuss central venous pressure (CVP) catheter and significance of findings. Central venous pressure is pressure within the superior vena cava, reflecting the pressure under which the blood is returned to the superior vena cava and right atrium. An informed consent is required because the procedure is invasive. For an accurate CVP measurement, a baseline must

be established for the transducer position. The zero point on the transducer needs to be at the level of the right atrium. The right atrium is located at the midaxillary line at the fourth intercostal space. The client must be supine and flat in bed for the most accurate reading. Normal CVP reading is 2–12 mm Hg. To get an accurate reading, place the client in a 45-degree position and the zero point of the transducer adjusted to the level of the right atrium. The client should be relaxed at the time of the measurements. A low CVP reading indicates fluid volume deficit, and a high CVP reading indicates fluid volume excess and the need for modification of fluid therapy.

7. **What complication could develop because of Mr. J's presenting symptoms on admission?** A complication that is most likely to develop with Mr. J because of his presenting symptoms is pulmonary edema (PE). Pulmonary edema develops when pulmonary interstitial fluid pressure rises from a negative range to a positive range causing rapid filling of the pulmonary interstitial spaces and alveoli. The most common causes of PE are left-sided heart failure, mitral valve disease, or damage to the pulmonary blood capillary membranes. Lethal PE can occur within minutes, depending on how high the capillary pressure rises. Crackles or rales in the lungs, S_3 heart sound, and pedal edema are indicators of fluid overload and the potential for the development of PE.

The following are prescribed:

- Digoxin (Lanoxin) 0.125 PO daily
- Captopril (Capoten) 12.5 mg PO three times per day
- Furosemide (Lasix) 80 mg IV stat, then 40 mg PO daily
- Spironolactone (Aldactone) 50 mg PO two times per day × five days
- Atenolol (Tenormin) 100 mg PO daily
- Diltiazem (Cardizem) 30 mg PO four times per day
- Nicotinic acid (Nicobid) 10 mg PO daily
- Rosiglitazone maleate (Avandia) 4 mg PO daily
- Docusate sodium (Colace) 100 mg PO three times per day

8. **What are the purposes for the prescribed orders?** *Digoxin* is a positive inotropic cardiac glycoside that slows and strengthens contractility of the heart muscle. This increases stroke volume and cardiac output and, in doing so, helps to decrease the workload of the heart and slow the progression of failure. It improves myocardial contractility, decreasing preload (the amount of fluid entering the chambers of the heart) and decreasing afterload (the amount of resistance or stretch the heart must use to deal with the excess fluid). When preload and afterload are decreased, contractility is improved and the heart is better able to empty blood from within the chambers. When the excess blood is emptied, stroke volume increases

and cardiac output is enhanced. With the enhancement of cardiac output, perfusion to the myocardium is enhanced and nutrients and oxygen are directed to the failing heart. The overall net effects of digoxin are improved stoke volume and cardiac output, improved renal perfusion, and prevention of fatal complications. *Captopril* is an angiotensin-converting enzyme (ACE) inhibitor antihypertensive agent used to reduced blood pressure. When captopril, digoxin, and diuretics are combined, functional capacity and hemodynamic parameters in clients with heart failure improve. Captopril reduces blood pressure by blocking the production of angiotensin II. Angiotensin II is a potent vasoconstrictor that stimulates hypertensive effects. When it is blocked by captopril's action, it produces vasodilation and, in doing so, reduces blood volume, preventing the effects of increased blood volume in the heart and blood vessels. Captopril reduces pulmonary congestion and peripheral edema by suppressing myocyte (a muscular tissue cell of the myocardium) growth. The suppression of myocytes reduces ventricular remodeling (change in shape and dimension of the ventricle) and helps in the stabilization of the heart. *Furosemide* is a potent loop diuretic that promotes diuresis. It is rapid acting and has antihypertensive properties. When given intravenously to a client with congested heart failure related to fluid congestion, furosemide acts quickly, within five minutes, to remove the congested fluid from the heart. Care must be taken to infuse no more than 20–40 mg/minute intravenous bolus to prevent rapid loss of fluid and hypotensive crisis. Furosemide functions by inhibiting sodium and chloride reabsorption primarily in Henle's loop and the proximal and distal renal tubules where these electrolytes are reabsorbed. Since about three-fourths of the sodium that remains after passage through the proximal tubule is absorbed in the ascending Henle's loop, diuretics that act on these sites can cause potent diuresis. Impairment of sodium reabsorption in Henle's loop causes a decrease in the osmolality of the interstitial fluid surrounding the collecting ducts and, in doing so, further impedes the kidney's ability to concentrate urine. Its antihypertensive properties decrease edema and intravascular volume, resulting in a decrease in workload of an already burdened heart. *Spironolactone* is a potassium-sparing diuretic that retains potassium in the serum. It is a potent diuretic and an electrolyte- and water-balance agent. Mr. J's K+ on admission is 3.0 (normal is 3.5–5 mEq). *Spironolactone* functions as a competitive antagonist to aldosterone and, in doing so, increases the loss of sodium in the urine while enhancing potassium retention, which helps maintain myocardial muscular tone. *Atenolol* is a beta-adrenergic blocking agent used to help lower blood pressure. It selectively blocks beta$_1$-adrenergic receptors located chiefly in cardiac muscle, and smooth muscle of bronchi and blood vessels. Its benefit for Mr. J is to selectively block beta$_1$ in the smooth muscle of blood vessels, resulting in a diminished sympathetic outflow from the vasomotor center in the brain to the peripheral blood vessels and an inhibition of renin release by the kidney. When the kidney inhibits renin release, there is a decrease in peripheral vascular resistance that lowers and stabilizes blood pressure. *Diltiazem* is a calcium channel-blocking agent that lowers arterial blood pressure and enhances myocardial blood flow. It dilates coronary arteries and peripheral arterioles, inhibits coronary artery spasm, and reduces total peripheral resistance (afterload), which helps improve myocardial blood flow by lowering arterial blood pressure at rest and during activities. *Nicotinic acid* is a form of niacin, a B-complex vitamin that helps to lower total cholesterol and triglyceride levels while increasing high-density lipoprotein (HDL) levels. It is a water-soluble vitamin that interferes with triglyceride synthesis and ultimately lowers hepatic secretion of very low density lipoprotein (VLDL) and decreases VLDL concentration, which leads to a reduction in circulating levels of LDL, with an overall net effect of lowering cholesterol concentration. Because nicotinic acid inhibits lipolysis in adipose tissue, it lowers the plasma concentration of free fatty acids, which usually are the main source of synthesis of triglycerides in the liver. *Rosiglitazone maleate* is a thiazolidinedione oral antidiabetic agent that lowers and stabilizes blood glucose by improving target cell response to insulin in type 2 diabetes. It has hormonal and antidiabetic properties that help to decrease cellular insulin resistance and decrease hepatic glucose output. *Docusate sodium* is a stool softener used to prevent constipation, which has a negative effect on the body especially in persons with cardiac problems. Docusate sodium acts to soften the stool with its detergent action that lowers surface tension, permitting water and fats to penetrate and soften stools for easier passage.

9. What are most common adverse reactions of the prescribed medications? The most common adverse reactions of *digoxin* are bradycardia, anorexia, nausea, vomiting, diarrhea, fatigue, and visual disturbances. Its most dangerous adverse effect is digoxin toxicity. The most common adverse reactions of **captopril** are first-dose hypotension, an irritating cough, chest pain, palpitations, tachycardia, and maculopapular rash. The most common adverse reactions of *furosemide* are hypokalemia, hyponatremia, dehydration, and hypochloremia. The most common adverse reactions of **atenolol** are bradycardia and hypotension. The most common adverse reactions of *diltiazem* are headache, bradycardia, AV block, hypotension, syncope, palpitations, and peripheral edema. The most common adverse reactions of *nicotinic acid* are transient headache, tingling of extremities, generalized flushing with sensation of warmth, pruritus, skin rash, and increased sebaceous gland activity. The most common adverse reaction of *rosiglitazone maleate* is fluid retention but can lead to cardiac failure, hypoglycemia, diarrhea, headache, fatigue, and anemia. The most

common adverse reaction of *ducosate sodium* is diarrhea, however dehydration and electrolyte imbalances may occur as a result of the increased loss of fluid and electrolytes through the stool.

10. Discuss the drug-to-drug and drug-to-food/herbal interactions of the prescribed medications? Drug-to-drug interactions may occur with the simultaneous use of *digoxin* and loop and thiazide diuretics, which may result in the increase of digoxin-induced dysrhythmias due to hypokalemia resulting from the diuresis. Angiotensin-converting enzymes (ACE) medications may increase potassium levels and thereby decrease the therapeutic responses of digoxin. Sympathomimetics such as dobutamine increase the heart rate, which would further increase the contractile force of the myocardial muscle, since that is one of the properties of digoxin. Simultaneous use of digoxin and dobutamine would therefore enhance tachydysrhythmias. Quinidine, if used simultaneously with digoxin, can cause the increase in plasma levels of digoxin, which would displace digoxin from tissue binding sites, reducing renal excretion of digoxin and resulting in increase risk for digoxin toxicity. The simultaneous use of verapamil, a calcium-channel blocker, can significantly increase plasma levels of digoxin and counteracts the benefits of digoxin. There are no clinically significant drug-to-food interactions established. Drug-to-herbal interactions may occur with the simultaneous use of hawthorn that contains natural cardiotonic ingredients. Hawthorn by itself increases the force of myocardial contraction and dilates blood vessels. The simultaneous use of hawthorn with digoxin increases the likelihood of toxic effects or the interference of the effectiveness of digoxin. If ginseng is taken simultaneously with digoxin or oral antidiabetic agents, it may cause an increase in hypoglycemia or increase in toxic effects. If cascara is taken simultaneously with digoxin, it may increase potassium loss and toxic effects of digoxin. Drug-to-drug interactions may occur with the simultaneous use of *captopril* and nitrates and antihypertensive medications that may enhance the hypotensive effects of captopril. Spironolactone and amiloride may increase the potassium levels if used simultaneously with captopril. Indomethacin may decrease the 24-hour antihypertensive effects of captopril, whereas probenecid may increase captopril blood levels due to decreased renal excretion. Drug-to-food interactions may occur if captopril is taken simultaneously with food. It should be taken 30–60 minutes before meals. There are no clinically significant drug-to-herbal interactions established. Drug-to-drug interactions may occur with the simultaneous use of *furosemide* and other diuretics and digoxin, which may increase the risk of toxicity due to the hypokalemic effects that may occur. Amphotericin B, if taken simultaneously with furosemide, may potentiate hypokalemia. The simultaneous use of furosemide and insulin may cause a blunting of hypoglycemic effects.

Charcoal decreases the absorption of furosemide from the gastrointestinal (GI) tract. Clofibrate enhances furosemide's diuretic action whereas hydantoins (phenytoin) decreases the diuretic effects. Use with propranolol may increase the serum plasma levels of propranolol. There are no clinically significant drug-to-food/herbal interactions established. The most common adverse reactions of *spironolactone* are confusion, headache, and dizziness. Drug-to-drug interactions may occur with the simultaneous use of ammonium chloride that may cause systemic acidosis. Drug-to-food interactions may occur with the simultaneous use of salt substitute, which may increase the risk of hyperkalemia. There are no clinically significant drug-to-herbal interactions established. With *atenolol*, drug-to-drug interactions occur with atropine and other anticholinergics that increase atenolol absorption from the GI tract. Nonsteroidal anti-inflammatory agents (NSAIDs) may decrease hypotensive effects and mask symptoms of hypoglycemia. Prazosin and terazocin may increase severe hypotensive response to the first dose of Atenolol. There are no clinically significant drug-to-food interactions established. Drug-to-herbal interactions may occur with the simultaneous use of hawthorn, which may potentiate the action of atenolol and alter the serum level. With *diltiazem HcL* drug-to-drug interactions may occur with the simultaneous use of beta-blockers, which may have additive effects on the AV node conduction and cause prolongation of the AV node response. The simultaneous use of digoxin or quinidine may increase digoxin or quinidine levels, and the simultaneous use with cimetidine may increase diltiazem serum levels and increase toxicity. Use with amiodarone may cause cardiotoxicity and with lithium increases the risk of neurotoxicity. Diltiazem will increase the serum levels of the following drugs: amiodipine, buspirone, cyclosporine, HMG-CoA reductase inhibitors, moricizine, cirolimus, tacrolimus, and theophyllines. There are no clinically significant drug-to-herbal interactions established. Drug-to-drug interactions may occur with the simultaneous use of *nicotinic acid* and antihypertensive agents by increasing the vasodilating effects of these agents. Nicotinic acid may decrease the effects of chenodial, probenecid, and sulfinpyrazone and increase the risk of myopathy and rhabdomyolysis is used with HMG-CoA reductase inhibitors. Drug-to-food interactions may occur with the simultaneous use of flaxseed, which may cause increase flushing. There are no clinically significant drug-to-herb interactions established. With *rosiglitazone maleate* drug-to-drug interactions may occur with the simultaneous use of insulin, which may increase the risk of heart failure or edema. Drug-to-food interactions may occur with the simultaneous use of garlic and ginseng, which may potentiate hypoglycemic effects. Drug-to-herbal interactions may occur with the simultaneous use of bittermelon with rosiglitazone, which may increase the risk of hypoglycemia. Finally, *ducosate sodium* may increase the absorption of mineral oil from the GI tract is used simultaneously with this agent. Otherwise, there are no clinically significant drug-to-drug or drug-to food/herbal interactions established.

11. Discuss specific nursing focus for the older client with heart failure. Specific nursing focus for older clients with heart failure requires close assessment. The lungs should be auscultated carefully while understanding that dependent crackles (rales) may not be an indication of heart failure in older adults. The nurse should not expect crackles to clear rapidly after medication administration because crackles may remain in the bases of the lungs over extended periods of time. Because clients with heart failure are usually on digoxin, and the older client's glomerular filtration rate is decreased, digoxin toxicity may develop. Therefore, the nurse should observe for manifestations of toxicity. If loop diuretics are administered monitoring for signs of excessive diuresis, dehydration, and hypokalemia should be implemented. Orthostatic hypotension also is a common finding in older clients receiving drug therapy for heart failure. A common complaint indicating possibly orthostatic hypotension is dizziness.

12. What are the major areas of home care assessment that are reimbursable by Medicare and other third-party payers?

- Assessing for signs of heart failure. Signs of heart failure are evidenced with activity intolerance, which requires self-care assistance and energy management. Assessing functional ability requires initial ongoing nursing supervision. Fatigue often alters functional ability, which would need environmental management or supervision upon discharge to home.
- Assessing nutritional status.
- Assessing home environment to determine the need for supervision or reinforcing safe environmental management while at home.
- Assessing the client's compliance and understanding of illness and its treatment and to reinforce the client's understanding of discharge protocol and temporarily monitor compliance with discharge instructions.
- Assessing the client's and caregiver coping skills, and make modifications where needed to avoid delay in rehabilitation.

13. Discuss client education and discharge planning for Mr. J. The nurse first needs to assess Mr. J's current level of knowledge related to his health condition. From there, the nurse should instruct him to avoid risk factors for exacerbating his heart failure by regaining and maintaining control of his diabetes, stopping smoking, and following his prescribed diet. He should be informed of the importance of adequate fluid intake when taking vasodilating agents to help maintain circulating volume and prevent hypotension. He needs optimum rest daily. He needs to know the signs and symptoms of adverse effects of his medications as well as the prescribed dosage and frequency for taking his medications. The importance of consulting with primary health care provider before using over-the-counter or herbal medications with the prescribed medications must be stressed as well as the importance of maintaining follow-up care with his primary health care provider. He needs to receive information regarding any referrals that his health care provider may have made, including the names of the contact people and their phone numbers.

References

Broyles, B. E. (2005). *Medical-Surgical Nursing Clinical Companion*. Durham, NC: Carolina Academic Press.

Corbet, J. V. (2004). *Laboratory Tests and Diagnostic Procedures with Nursing Diagnoses* (6th ed.). Upper Saddle River, NJ: Prentice Hall.

Gahart, B. L. and Nazareno, A. R. (2005). *2005 Intravenous Medications*. St. Louis: Mosby.

Guyton, A. C. and Hall, J. E. (2006). *Textbook of Medical Physiology* (11th ed.). Philadelphia: W. B. Saunders.

Huether, S. E. and McCance, K. L. (2006). *Understanding Pathophysiology* (3rd ed.). St. Louis: Mosby.

Ignatavicius, D. D. and Workman, M. L. (2006). *Medical-Surgical Nursing across the Health Care Continuum* (5th ed.). Philadelphia: W. B. Saunders.

Kuhn, M. A. (April 2002). "Herbal Remedies: Drug-Herb Interactions." *Critical Care Nurse* 22(2): 22–30.

Lehne, R. A. (2003). *Pharmacology for Nursing Care* (5th ed.). Philadelphia: W. B. Saunders.

Spratto, G. R. and Woods, A. L. (2005). *2005 Edition: PDR Nurse's Drug Handbook*. Clifton Park, NY: Thomson Delmar Learning.

Perineal Abscess and Cellulitis of a Lower Extremity

GENDER

F

AGE

65

SETTING

- Hospital

ETHNICITY

- Black American

PREEXISTING CONDITIONS

COEXISTING CONDITIONS

- Obesity
- Diabetes

LIFESTYLE

- Self-employed hair designer

COMMUNICATION

DISABILITY

- Activity intolerance

SOCIOECONOMIC STATUS

- Low

SPIRITUAL/RELIGIOUS

- Nondenominational

PHARMACOLOGIC

- Glyburide (Diabeta)
- Metformin (Glucophage)
- Ampicillin sodium/sulbactam sodium (Unasyn)

PSYCHOSOCIAL

- Anxiety

LEGAL

ETHICAL

ALTERNATIVE THERAPY

- Ginger, garlic

PRIORITIZATION

- Infection control

DELEGATION

- RN
- CNA
- Client education

MODERATE

THE CARDIOVASCULAR AND LYMPHATIC SYSTEMS

Level of difficulty: Moderate

Overview: This case involves a thorough assessment of the client's condition, including the client's medical history. The nurse must use clinical experience and critical thinking to provide safe and effective care while prioritizing and implementing independent and dependent functions. Once the client is assessed by the nurse, the nursing assistant can be assigned to assist the client with hygiene care. The nursing assistant is instructed to observe and report to the nurse any changes of the skin.

Client Profile

Ms. V is a 65-year-old female, a self-employed hair stylist, who is accompanied to the hospital by her adult daughter. Ms. V is referred to the hospital by her primary health care provider to be evaluated for a perineal abscess and cellulitis of the left lower extremity. Ms. V is 5′4″ and weighs 250 pounds.

Case Study

Ms. V is a re-admission to this hospital. She was previously admitted for an ulcerated great toe of the right foot. Her primary reason for admission today is for a perineal abscess and cellulitis of the left lower extremity. Ms V's arms and legs are large, and her abdomen is large and pendulous. She is alert and oriented to all stimuli and is able to provide significant information during the nursing history and assessment, but she reports discomfort at her buttocks and her left lower extremity on movement. Ms. V denies exercise but admits to compliance with her medication regimen. She brings the prescribed medication, glyburide/metformin, which she reports taking twice daily, and metoclopramine, which she reports taking twice a day and at night. Her past medical history (PMH) reveals NIDDM for 20 years and peripheral vascular disease with recurrent cellulitis for five years. On physical assessment her vital signs are:

Blood pressure: 130/72
Pulse: 80 and regular
Respirations: 18
Temperature: 101.4° F

Her left leg is swollen with erythema of the left toes present and an unusual odor, although there is no open wound. Peripheral pulses of bilateral lower extremities are positive (+2) with the exception of the popliteal and dorsalis pedis of the left foot that is not assessed due to the cellulitis. There is erythema and swelling of the calf of the left lower extremity; the area is tender to touch. Ms. V reports nausea and vomiting for the past 24 hours, which she cannot relate to any specific cause. She reports monitoring of her serum glucose four times per day before meals with a glucometer and reports the most recent reading of 180 mg/dL. Ms. V informs the nurse that she noticed the glucose remained elevated at 180 mg/dL, but on two occasions it was 200 mg/dL. She also states that the glucose elevations were during the time she had the pain and redness of the extremity and unusual pain and odor from her perineal area. Admission labs are:

White blood cell (WBC) count: 13,000/mm^3
Glucose: 176 mg/dL

Hematocrit (Hct): 38%
Hemoglobin (Hgb): 14 g/dL
Platelet count (PLT): 1,600,000/mm^3
Sodium (Na): 132 mEq/L
Potassium (K+): 4.8 mEq/L
Calcium: 9 mg/dL
Blood urea nitrogen (BUN): 18 mg/dL
Creatinine: 2 mg/dL
Urinalysis (U/A): negative for abnormalities
Phosphorous: 3.7 mg/dL
Albumin: 3 mg/dL

Ms. V is seen by the health care provider for a complete history and physical. Ms. V is assigned to bed rest with bathroom privileges, but her left leg is to be elevated on a pillow when sitting or in bed. A registered dietitian visits with Ms. V, and a nutritional plan is designed for her. MRI of left lower extremity reveals soft tissue inflammation of the foot and generalized infection of the deeper connective tissue, and Doppler studies are positive for peripheral pulses in bilateral lower extremities except the pedal and dorsalis pedis pulses, which are weak. Culture and sensitivity of the perineal abscess reveal E. coli of the wound; gram stain reveals gram-positive cocci.

Questions

1. What are common nursing diagnoses for clients with perineal abscess and lower extremity cellulitis?

2. What major complications may develop due to perineal abscess and lower extremity cellulitis?

3. What types of ulcers are most likely to develop due to the client's disease processes and the altered immobility?

4. What are some pressure management strategies that may be used to facilitate healing of perineal abscess and cellulitis of the lower extremity?

5. Discuss the importance of nutritional status maintenance for clients with alteration in skin integrity.

6. What are the two steps of a pressure ulcer prevention program?

7. What are some noninvasive measures the nurse may use to prevent prolonged contact of the skin with urinary substances?

8. What are the purposes for the prescribed orders?

9. What are the most common adverse reactions of the prescribed medications?

10. Discuss the drug-to-drug, drug-to-food/herbal interactions for the prescribed medications.

11. Discuss nursing implications related to risk for pressure ulcers and alteration in skin integrity.

Questions and Suggested Answers

1. What are common nursing diagnoses for clients with perineal abscess and lower extremity cellulitis?

- Acute pain or chronic pain R/T skin trauma and wound infection
- Impaired tissue integrity R/T to perineal abscess and cellulitis
- Risk for infection R/T disease process
- Hyperthermia R/T hypermetabolic rate
- Risk for injury R/T adverse effects of medications
- Deficient knowledge R/T condition, treatment, home care

2. What major complications may develop due to perineal abscess and lower extremity cellulitis? A major complication that may develop due to the perineal abscess is ascending infection of the genitourinary system. A major complication that may develop due to the cellulitis of the lower extremity is ulceration of the extremity. Bacteremia and sepsis may develop if the perineal wound is not aggressively treated, if the client becomes severely immunocompromised, or if local blood supply to the wound is impaired.

3. What types of ulcers are most likely to develop due to the client's disease processes and the altered immobility? Ulcers are most likely to develop because this client will be immobilized in a supine position for prolonged periods of time. Decubitus ulcer is one of the ulcers that could develop because of the history of diabetes mellitus, which complicates the circulatory system and enhances the development of ulcer formation. In diabetes mellitus, there is increased blood sugar that impairs blood flow and the release of needed oxygen. There are usually impaired local immune and cell defenses that could enhance ulcer formation. Vascular changes in lower extremities result in arteriosclerosis and eventually result in diabetes-induced arteriosclerosis, eventually leading to multiple occlusions with decreased blood flow to the lower extremities. Over a period of time, peripheral vascular disease and neuropathy predispose clients to development of diabetic ulcers. Altered immobility such as bed rest, especially in a supine position, can result in pressure ulcers. The unrelieved pressure, especially over bony prominence at the sacral area, is a good medium for the development of pressure ulcers. Consistent in areas such as the sacrum results in pressure that is greater than capillary pressure and arteriolar pressure, with occlusion of blood flow. If the pressure continues, platelets aggregate in the endothelial cells surrounding the capillaries and form microthrombi. The microthrombi impede blood flow, resulting in ischemia and hypoxia of tissues. The combination of interruption of blood flow and prolonged pressure to an area eventually results in stage II ulcer formation, such as abrasion, blister, or shallow crater. Cellulitis prolongs the inflammatory phase by inducing tissue protease degradation. When the

inflammatory phase is prolonged, tissue growth factors are impaired and this delays collagen deposition and healing. These factors would delay the healing of the perineal abscess, with resultant ulcer formation developing at the perineal area.

4. **What are some pressure management strategies that may be used to facilitate healing of perineal abscess and cellulitis of the lower extremity?**

- Use the Braden scale to predict pressure score risk. The scale assesses the sensory perception of the client to determine the client's ability to respond meaningfully to pressure-related discomfort. It looks at the moisture to determine the degree to which the skin is exposed. It looks at the degree of physical activity and mobility in regard to the client's ability to change and control body position. It looks at nutrition with focus on the client's usual food intake pattern and at factors that would enhance friction and shearing of the skin. Other tools for skin assessment include the Norton scale, the Gosnell scale, and the Knoll assessment tool.
- Assess the client carefully to determine the most appropriate support surface. Keep in mind that pressure-relieving devices reduce the interface pressure between the body and the support surface below 32 mm Hg, which is capillary closing pressure. Examples of pressure-relieving devices are air-fluidized bed (Clinitron Bed), low air-loss (The KinAir III) bed, eggcrate mattress, static air mattress (Roho Dry Flotation Mattress System), and alternating air mattress (Grant Dyna-CARE).
- Avoid applying pressure to the affected body parts to reduce the risk for skin breakdown by preventing excess pressure on areas of the body. To ensure pressure relief, follow a 24-hour training schedule (side to back to other side to supine). Encourage the client to shift from position if possible at least every 15 minutes.
- Monitor the client's nutritional intake because malnutrition is one of the major causes of alteration in skin integrity and ulcers. Nutritional intake for the client with risk for ulcers should include a balanced diet with sufficient proteins, carbohydrates, and vitamin C.

5. **Discuss the importance of nutritional status maintenance for clients with alteration in skin integrity.** Nutritional status maintenance of the client with skin integrity impairment is critical for wound healing, because intact skin and wound healing are dependent on a positive nitrogen balance and adequate serum protein. Deficits in nitrogen balance and serum protein delay wound healing, therefore, a registered dietitian or nutritionist should be a part of skin impairment reduction strategy that includes moisture barriers, scheduled repositioning, and balanced nutrition, which includes sufficient protein and vitamins such as C and zinc. Protein is needed in this

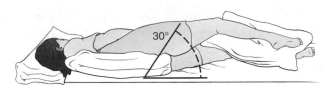

To avoid pressure points, position clients in the 30-degree lateral position.

case to repair body tissues. The significant role of vitamin C in tissue building is its ability to promote collagen, which enhances healing of wounds by holding tissues together. Zinc is effective in tissue repair because of its role in the functioning of the immune system, which is altered in diabetes mellitus and in problems of inflammation.

6.   What are the two steps of a pressure ulcer prevention program? The two steps of a pressure ulcer prevention program are identification of high-risk clients and the implementation of aggressive intervention for prevention with the use of pressure-relief and pressure-reduction products such as over-bed cradle, sheepskin, air-fluidized bed, eggcrate mattress, or alternating air mattress to reduce the interface pressure between the body and the support surface below 32 mm Hg.

7.   What are some noninvasive measures the nurse may use to prevent prolonged contact of the skin with urinary substances? Substances from urine include urea, bacteria, yeast, and enzymes and are irritants that can lead to skin breakdown. Daily inspection of the involved areas is a major noninvasive measure to prevent alteration in skin integrity impairment, to include: washing of the perineal area with a pH-balanced soap to maintain the normal acid level, avoiding massaging reddened areas so as to avoid damaging capillary beds, checking for incontinence at least hourly, and changing soiled clothing and bed linen frequently to prevent skin irritation.

The following are prescribed:

- Acetaminophen (Tylenol) 650 mg PO q6hrs for temp greater than 101°, and notify MD
- Ampicillin sodium/sulbactam sodium (Unasyn) IV 1g q6h
- Glyburide (Diabeta) 2.5 mg/metformin (Glucophage) 500 mg PO two times per day
- Metoclopramide (Reglan) 10 mg PO four times per day and at bedtime
- 2,000-calorie American Diabetic Association (ADA) diet
- Fingerstick glucose q shift; notify MD for glucose above 180 mg/dL
- Perineal wound care with normal saline wet-to-dry dressing

8.   What are the purposes for the prescribed orders? *Acetaminophen* is a non-opioid analgesic and antipyretic used in this case to lower elevation of

temperature, which if elevated would increase the client's metabolic rate and compound present problems. It inhibits the effects of pyrogens on the hypothalamic heat-regulation system. *Ampicillin sodium/sulbactam sodium* is a penicillin antibiotic used to treat gram-negative and gram-positive organisms. It irreversibly inhibits beta lactamases, and the sulbactam additive broadens the antibiotic activity especially with organisms that may be resistant to ampicillin alone. It helps to stabilize the disease processes because of its bactericidal property that eradicates organisms from invaded sites. Because it is effective in its broad-spectrum activity, it will help to hasten the healing of the perineal abscess and the cellulitic leg by eradicating varied types of organisms. *Glyburide*, in combination with *metformin* as antidiabetic agents, is to enhance the function of the pancreas and the beta cells as a unit. *Glyburide* lowers blood sugar concentration by sensitizing functioning pancreatic beta cells to release more insulin in the presence of elevated serum glucose levels. *Metformin* suppresses gluconeogenesis and hepatic production of glucose and, in doing so, lowers glucose levels. Because both drugs stabilize glucose concentration, the pancreas can function normally, and false elevation of glucose, exposing the client to hyperglycemic effects, will not occur. *Metoclopramide* is a gastrointestinal (GI) stimulant that increases stomach emptying time and has the ability to increase the resting tone of the esophagus sphincter and the tone and amplitude of upper-GI contractions. As a result, gastric emptying and intestinal transit are accelerated with little effect on gastric, biliary, or pancreatic secretions. *Metoclopramide* is also prescribed as prophylaxis for gastropareisis, which usually develops in persons with diabetes mellitus. Its specific anti-emetic effect occurs from drug-induced elevation of the chemoreceptor trigger zone (CTZ) threshold and, in doing so, enhances gastric emptying and relieves nausea and vomiting. A *2,000-calorie ADA diet* is to help reduce the client's weight, which will help control diabetes. Another purpose for the 2,000-calorie ADA diet is to prevent her pancreas from having to produce insulin in excess, which could eventually result in type 1 diabetes mellitus. *Fingerstick glucose* is to monitor glucose levels that may fluctuate in lieu of the cellulitis that is an additional physiologic stress to the body and can cause the release of glycogenic hormones in the body and further increase glucose levels. If the glucose reaches 180 mg/dl, this is an indication that the pancreas beta cells are not functioning optimally to produce endogenous insulin, and therefore exogenous insulin is needed to prevent complications. Fingerstick glucose monitoring provides immediate feedback that helps providers tailor management strategies, such as dietary changes, modification of oral agents, and implication of insulin therapy if needed. Consistently elevated blood glucose levels can result in macrovascular changes, therefore monitoring of blood glucose levels is a significant component of diabetic management. Macrovascular changes that commonly occur with consistently elevated blood glucose levels include coronary artery disease, cerebrovascular disease, peripheral vascular disease, and hypertension. Macrovascular disease of large arteries reflects atherosclerosis with deposits of lipids within the inner layer of vessel walls. These clients are known to have more anginal (chest pain) and higher mortality with myocardial infarction (MI). Cardiomyopathy may occur secondary to small vessel infarctions causing myocardial fibrosis and hypertrophy. Atherothromboembolic infarctions (transient ischemic attacks) and cerebral vascular accidents may occur due to fatty deposits breaking off from inner vessel walls and traveling to areas of the brain. Transient ischemic attacks or cerebrovascular accidents may also occur due to impaired circulation promoting blood clots, which may travel to areas of the brain, resulting in transient ischemic attacks and cerebral vascular accidents. The incidence of carotid bruits, intermittent claudication, absent pedal pulses, and ischemic gangrene is increased in diabetes mellitus. Peripheral vascular disease and neuropathy augment the morbidity associated with trauma and infection in the lower extremity. An increased rate of hypertension has been noted in the diabetic population, and hypertension is a major risk factor for stroke and nephropathy. *Perineal wound care* with normal saline wet-to-dry sterile dressing is done to aid in healing. Normal saline solution is the preferred cleansing agent because it is physiologically compatible, does not harm tissue, and adequately cleanses most tissue. The wet dressing directly adheres to the wound and helps with debridement, and the dry sterile dressing aids in absorbing drainage or exudate.

9. What are the most common adverse reactions of the prescribed medications? Common adverse reactions of *acetaminophen* are rare, but hepatotoxicity may occur in persons who are alcoholics or in the event an excess dose is consumed. The most common adverse reactions for *ampicillin sodium/sulbactam sodium* are rash, itching, pain at injection site (if infused too rapidly), diarrhea, and nausea. Clients with allergies to penicillin are at risk for anaphylactic reactions to ampicillin sodium. The most common adverse reactions of *glyburide* are hypoglycemia, heartburn, and nausea. The most common adverse reactions of *metformin* are nausea, vomiting, abdominal pain, bitter or metallic taste, diarrhea, bloating, and anorexia. The most common adverse reactions of *metoclopramide* are restlessness, drowsiness, and diarrhea.

10. Discuss the drug-to-drug and drug-to-food/herbal interactions of the prescribed medications? When using *acetaminophen* drug-to-drug interactions may occur with the simultaneous use of cholestyramine, which may decrease acetaminophen absorption. The simultaneous use of carbamazepine, phenytoin, barbiturates, propranolol, rifampin, sulfinpyrazone, and isoniazid may increase the potential for hepatotoxicity. Use with nonsteroidal anti-inflammatory agents (NSAIDs) increase the risk of hypertension in women, and use with oral contraceptives increases biotransformation of acetaminophen in the liver, decreasing its half-life. *Acetaminophen* decreases the serum levels of lamotrigine and zidovudine, thus decreasing the effectiveness of these agents. Milk thistle helps prevent acetaminophen hepatotoxicity. Drug-to-drug interactions may occur with the simultaneous use of *ampicillin sodium/sulbactam sodium* and allopurinol, which may increase the incidence of rash. Oral contraceptives may reduce bactericidal effects of ampicillin. There are no clinically significant drug-to-food/herbal interactions established. Drug-to-drug interactions may occur with the simultaneous use of glyburide and alcohol or drugs with alcohol ingredients. The use of alcohol may cause disulfiram-like reactions. Oral anticoagulant, chloramphenicol, clofibrate, and cimetidine also cause drug interactions by increasing or decreasing glyburide levels. Drug-to-food/herbal interactions may occur with the simultaneous use of ginseng and garlic that may increase hypoglycemic effects. Drug-to-drug interactions may occur with the simultaneous use of *metformin HcL* and captopril, furosemide, or nifedipine, which increase metformin effect and may cause hypoglycemia responses. Cimetidine may cause a reduction in metformin's clearance from the body, which may increase toxicity. Iodinated contrast media increases the risk of acute renal failure and lactic acidosis. Drug-to-food/herbal interactions may occur with the simultaneous use of ginseng and garlic that may increase hypoglycemic effects. With *metoclopramide* drug-to-drug interactions are seen with the simultaneous use of central nervous system (CNS) depressant agents that may increase sedating effects. Anticholinergic agents such as atropine may antagonize GI motility. Use with cimetidine, digoxin, and narcotic analgesics decreases the effects of these medications. An increased release of catecholamines occurs with simultaneous use with monoamine oxidase (MAO) inhibitors. Concurrent use with CNS depressants, succinylcholine, cyclosporine, acetaminophen, or tetracyclines increase the serum levels of these agents and can lead to toxicity. There are no clinically significant drug-to-food/herbal interactions established.

11. Discuss nursing implications related to risk for pressure ulcers and alteration in skin integrity. Although on the surface prevention by using pressure-reduction devices such as air-fluidized bed, low air-loss bed, eggcrate mattress, static air mattress, alternating air mattress, high protein diets, and appropriate dressing materials appear expensive, the actual cost in nursing hours when caring for a client with even one pressure ulcer is far more costly. Nurses need to remain cognizant of the legislation signed in 1999 that allows prevention costs as well as care costs to be justly reimbursed and, therefore, consider aggressively implementing care for all stages of pressure ulcer prevention in care setting as a priority.

References

Black, J. M. and Hawks, J. H. (2005). *Medical-Surgical Nursing: Clinical Management for Positive Outcomes* (7th ed.). St. Louis: Mosby.

Broyles, B. E. (2005). *Medical-Surgical Nursing Clinical Companion*. Durham, NC: Carolina Academic Press.

Corbet, J. V. (2004). *Laboratory Tests and Diagnostic Procedures with Nursing Diagnoses* (6th ed.). Upper Saddle River, NJ: Prentice Hall.

Gahart, B. L. and Nazareno, A. R. (2005). *2005 Intravenous Medications*. St. Louis: Mosby.

Harkreader, H. and Hogan, M. A. (2004). *Fundamentals of Nursing: Caring and Clinical Judgment* (2nd ed.). Philadelphia: W. B. Saunders.

Huether, S. E. and McCance, K. L. (2004). *Understanding Pathophysiology* (3rd ed.). St. Louis: Mosby.

Ignatavicius, D. D. and Workman, M. L. (2005). *Medical-Surgical Nursing across the Health Care Continuum* (5th ed.). Philadelphia: W. B. Saunders.

Lewis, S. M., Heitkemper, M. M., and Dirksen, S. R. (2003). *Medical-Surgical Nursing: Assessment and Management of Clinical Problems* (6th ed.). St. Louis: Mosby.

Spratto, G. R. and Wood, A. L. (2005). *2005 Edition: PDR Nurse's Drug Handbook*. Clifton Park, NY: Thomson Delmar Learning.

PART FOUR

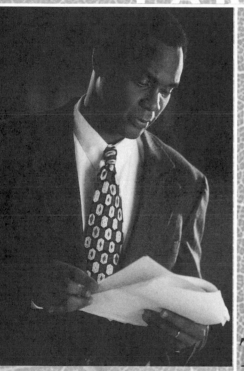

The Nervous System

CASE STUDY 1

Migraine Headache

GENDER

F

AGE

43

SETTING

■ Health care provider's office

ETHNICITY/ CULTURE

■ Black American

PREEXISTING CONDITIONS

COEXISTING CONDITIONS

■ Hypertension

LIFESTYLE

■ Director, LPN program

COMMUNICATION

DISABILITY

SOCIOECONOMIC STATUS

■ Middle

SPIRITUAL/RELIGIOUS

■ Baptist

PHARMACOLOGIC

■ Metoprolol tartrate (Lopressor)
■ Sumatriptan succinate (Imitrex)

PSYCHOSOCIAL

■ Anxiety
■ Depression

LEGAL

ETHICAL

ALTERNATIVE THERAPY

■ Gingko

PRIORITIZATION

■ Relieve pain

DELEGATION

■ RN
■ Client education

THE NERVOUS SYSTEM

Level of difficulty: Easy

Overview: This case involves a thorough assessment of the client's condition, including all drugs and/or herbals that she is currently taking. It also involves detailed medication history to get insight into the client's overall health status. Because headache is often the presenting symptom of various physiologic and psychological disturbances, a general health history should be an essential component of the client's data base.

Client Profile

Mrs. Z is a 43-year-old registered nurse (RN) and the director of a Career Ladder Nursing Program at a university. The program is a one-year program and has had a high percentage of enrollments for the past 12 years, with a consistent 90% pass rate on the PN-NCLEX exam. However, over the past four years, the program has had rapid turnover of faculty, needing frequent faculty replacement at a time when the PN-NCLEX exam is modified for higher critical thinking, delegation, and application. Mrs. Z believes that "these factors are triggers for stress and headache she is experiencing."

Case Study

Mrs. Z is seen in her primary health care provider's office with complaints of periodic and recurrent attacks of severe headaches. Her vital signs during assessment reveal:

Blood pressure: 150/90
Pulse: 60
Respirations: 18
Temperature: 98.6° F

She is 5'9" and weighs 200 pounds. During the gathering of data, Mrs. Z reports history of hypertension and takes norvasc (Amlodipine) 10 mg PO daily and hydrochlorothiazide (HydroDIURIL) 25 mg PO daily. The nurse questions Mrs. Z about her sleep patterns, which she reports have been altered over the past three months with only short periods of sleep (two hours) before awakening. She denies any known family history of headaches or family stressors. Mrs. Z is seen by the health care provider for further history and assessment. She reports migraine attacks that occur three or four days per month and states she has had headaches for several years, but not as severe as the ones that cause her to seek medical intervention. After discussion of the presenting problem (headache) and reviewing of the nursing history, a routine assessment is done and a diagnosis of migraine headache is made. Mrs. Z is given a three-month appointment for reevaluation and a prescription for medications.

Questions

1. Discuss the different phases of migraine headaches.

2. How is the diagnosis of migraine headache determined?

3. What are common nursing diagnoses for clients with migraine headache?

4. Pain management is the *priority* care for the client with migraine headache. What are the two types of therapy used to accomplish this priority?

5. What are the purposes for the prescribed orders?

Questions (continued)

6. What are the most common adverse reactions, drug-to-drug, drug-to-food/herbal interactions for the prescribed medications?

7. Discuss the complementary and alternative therapies currently used for migraine headaches.

8. Discuss food triggers for migraine headaches.

9. Discuss some commonly used herbs for the prevention of migraine headaches.

10. Discuss client education for migraine headaches.

Questions and Suggested Answers

1. **Discuss the different phases of migraine headaches.** Migraine headaches are subdivided by the International Headache Society (IHS) into those *with aura* (formerly called classic migraine) and those *without aura* (formerly called common migraine). *Migraine with aura* involves at lease three of the following: (1) reversible aura that involves brain dysfunction; (2) aura symptoms that develop gradually over more than four minutes, or two or more symptoms occurring in succession; (3) no aura lasting more than 60 minutes; (4) headache that follows aura within 60 minutes. Migraine with aura occurs in only 10% of migraine episodes. It is sharply defined and may last for 10–30 minutes before the start of the headache and may include sensory dysfunction (e.g., visual field defects, tingling or burning sensations, paresthesias), motor dysfunction (e.g., weakness, paralysis), dizziness, confusion, and even loss of consciousness. The classic aura symptom is perception of flashing lights in one quadrant of the visual field, often termed scintillating scotomata. Migraine with aura usually occurs when there is significant vasoconstriction that reduces cerebral blood flow. However, no permanent deficits usually result from the cerebral reduction because the vasoconstriction is predominantly unilateral. The form of the aura that the client experiences is dependent on the area of the brain affected. Migraine with aura usually peaks in one hour and may last several hours. *Migraine without aura* involves at least two of the following characteristics: unilateral location, pulsating quality, moderate to severe intensity, worsening with activity, and at least one of either (1) nausea and vomiting or (2) photophobia and phonophobia. Migraine without aura is the most common type of migraine headache, and the headache itself may last several hours or days. Clinical manifestations that might occur in migraine with or without aura are generalized edema, irritability, pallor, nausea and vomiting, and sweating.

2. **How is the diagnosis of migraine headache determined?** The diagnosis of migraine headache is based on the client's history and physical and neurologic assessment. Neuroimaging such as magnetic resonance imaging

(MRI) may be indicated if the client has other neurologic findings, a history of seizures, findings not consistent with a migraine, or a change in the severity or symptoms of frequency of attacks. Brain scan, electroencephalogram, skull, and cervical spine X-rays may be used to determine potential cause(s) for the headaches. If psychogenic headaches are suspected, the interdisciplinary team may consider a referral for a complete psychiatric evaluation.

3. What are common nursing diagnoses for clients with migraine headache?
   - Acute pain R/T headache
   - Anxiety R/T lack of knowledge about headache's etiology and ways to treat
   - Hopelessness R/T chronic pain, alteration of lifestyle, and ineffective treatment modalities

4. Pain management is the *priority* care for the client with migraine headache. Which are the two types of therapy used to accomplish this priority? ***Abortive drug therapy*** is aimed at alleviating pain during the aura phase (if present) or soon after the headache has started. Medications used with abortive therapy include analgesic such as acetaminophen (Tylenol), which may be administered for mild to moderate headache. However, if acetaminophen does not relieve the headache, ergotamine (Ergomar)

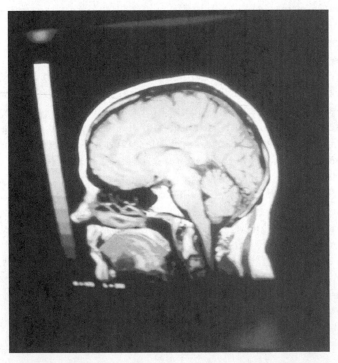

Neuroimaging such as magnetic resonance imaging (MRI) may be a useful neurologic assessment in diagnosing migraine headaches.

will be implemented. Ergotamine relieves the headache by inhibiting the reuptake of norepinephrine into postganglionic nerve terminals of the sympathetic nervous system. This allows more norepinephrine to attach to alpha-adrenergic sites on smooth muscle in the artery wall, thereby causing prolonged vasoconstriction of cranial blood vessels. Selected serotonin receptors such as those classified as "triptans" are used to treat the pathologic process of migraine. One such drug is sumatriptan (Imitrex). It relieves the headache by reducing neurogenic inflammation of the cerebral blood vessels and producing vasoconstriction. Sumatriptam not only aborts an ongoing migraine attack, but it relieves both headache and the associated symptoms such as nausea, photophobia, and phonophobia. Triptans should be taken at the first symptom of migraine headache. Muscle relaxants such as diazepam (Valium) may be prescribed to decrease muscle spasms that may occur with the headache. *Preventive therapy* includes counseling to alter coping mechanisms and modification of behavior or altering of stressors. The use of antidepressants may also be prescribed for preventive therapy. Amitriptyline (Elavil), a tricyclic antidepressant, may be prescribed. Amitryptyline works to relieve depression by blocking serotonin receptors in the central and peripheral nervous system, thus blocking the reuptake of norepinephrine and serotonin by nerve endings so that these transmitters remain active for longer periods of time after secretion, resulting in the reversing of the depression. It is presumed that the norepinephrine and serotonin systems normally provide drive to the limbic areas of the brain to increase a person's sense of well-being and create happiness.

The following are prescribed:

- Metoprolol tartrate (Lopressor) 50 mg PO two times per day
- Sumatriptan succinate (Imitrex) 100 mg PO as soon as migraine symptoms appear

5. What are the purposes for the prescribed orders? *Metoprolol tartrate* is a beta$_1$ adrenergic blocking agent that lowers blood pressure by inhibiting the action of beta$_1$ receptor cells in the heart and brain that control the dilation of blood vessels, which is thought to be the major function with migraine headaches. *Sumatriptan succinate* is an antimigraine agent and a "selective agonist for a vascular 5-HT receptor located in the cranial arteries, the basilar artery, and the vasculative of the dura mater" (Spratto and Woods, 1158). It causes vasoconstriction and consequently relieves migraine headaches that are caused by vasodilation of these vessels.

6. What are the most common adverse reactions, drug-to-drug, drug-to-food-herbal interactions for the prescribed medications? The most common adverse reactions of *metoprolol tartrate* are dizziness, hypotension, fatigue, weakness, insomnia, impotence, bradycardia, heartburn, and shortnesss of breath. Drug-to-drug interactions may occur with the simultaneous use of barbiturates and rifampin, which may decrease the effects of *metoprolol tartrate*. The simultaneous use of cimetidine, quinidine, or propylthiouracil may increase effects of metoprolol tartrate. The simultaneous use of indomethacin may attenuate hypotensive response, and IV phenytoin and verapamil may increase the risk of heart block and bradycardia. The simultaneous use with nitrates or antihypertensive agents may increase hypotension. Concurrent use with cocaine, ephedrine, epinephrine, norepinephrine, phenylephrine, or pseudoephedrine may cause unopposed alpha-adrenergic stimulation (excessive hypertension and bradycardia). Diphenhydramine, methimazole, phenobarbital, propylthiouracil, and rifampin decrease the effects of metoprolol tartrate. Concurrent use with insulin or oral hypoglycemic agents may alter their effectiveness. There are no clinically significant drug-to-food/herbal interactions established. The most common adverse effects of *sumatriptan succinate* occur with subcutaneous and oral administration of the agent. These include flushing, hypertension, bradycardia, tachycardia, palpitations, syncope, fatigue, dizziness, vertigo, and drowsiness. Serious adverse effects may occur, including life-threatening dysrrythmias (atrial and ventricular fibrillation, ventricular tachycardia, myocardial infarction, and ischemic ST elevations). These symptoms are common in persons with a cardiovascular disease history or those that exceed the safe dose of sumatriptan succinate, or they may occur as idiosyncratic responses. No more than 200 mg should be taken in a 24-hour period. Drug-to-drug interactions may occur with the simultaneous use of ergot drugs, including prolonging vasospastic reactions, monoamine oxidase (MAO) inhibitors that increase the half-life of sumatriptan, and selective serotonin reuptake inhibitors that may cause weakness, hyperreflexia, and incoordination, although these reactions are rare. Although many food triggers have been identified as causes of migraines, there are no drug-to-food interactions established.

7. Discuss the complementary and alternative therapies currently used for migraine headaches. *Biofeedback* is an alternative therapy used with migraine headache. In biofeedback the client is taught to control an involuntary function through the use of monitors. The client learns both muscle relaxation and blood-vessel relaxation methods, because many clients have combination-type headaches. *Self-hypnosis* has been documented as an aid to relief migraine headache. Self-hypnosis is the ability to tap the healing potential of the human mind. It allows the client to give him or herself helpful suggestions to aid with relaxation of the mind and body. It also expands and builds on the self-awareness that is developing through the use of imagery and meditative relaxation states.

8. Discuss food triggers for migraine headaches. Some foods such as chocolate, cheese, citrus fruits, coffee, and pork contain substances that may

trigger migraine headaches. For instance, tyramine, an amine found in foods, is believed to cause migraine headache. Dietary tyramine is absorbed from the intestine, transported to the liver, and then immediately inactivated by the hepatic MAO. In the presence of MAO, inhibition of neuronal raises the levels of norepinephrine in sympathetic nerve terminals; inhibition of hepatic MAO also allows dietary tyramine to pass through the liver and enter the systemic circulation in an intact form. However, upon reaching peripheral sympathetic nerve terminals, tyramine promotes the release of accumulated norepinephrine stores, which triggers abnormal response of the sympathetic nervous system, resulting in excessive stimulation of the heart and massive vasoconstriction. The excessive stimulation of the heart and the massive vasoconstriction decreases cerebral blood flow to the cerebral vessels, resulting in the occurrence of a headache. Another pharmacological agent in food that has been linked to migraine is the vasoactive amine phenylethylamine, which is found in chocolate and has the same mechanism as that of tyramine. It is also believed that monosodium glutamate (MSG), a naturally occurring salt of glutamic acid, which if taken in excess (Chinese restaurant syndrome) can cause temporary vasoconstriction of blood vessels, resulting in alteration of cerebral blood flow and headache.

9. Discuss some commonly used herbs for the prevention of migraine headaches. Although further research is needed to determine the benefits of herbs as alternative therapy for migraine headaches, a number of herbs are currently being used by some consumers to treat migraines. Some of these are feverfew (Tanacetum parthenium), bay (Laurus nobilis), willow (Salix), ginger (Zingiber officinate), red pepper (Capsicum), lemon balm (Melissa officinsalis), and purslane (Portulaca oleracea).

10. Discuss client education for migraine headaches. The client should be provided with a list of foods and beverages that contain tyramine and be instructed on the importance to avoid them. Foods and beverages that contain tyramine include alcoholic drinks such as beer, wine, and hard liquor. Foods that should be considered possible triggers in the development of migraine headache include aged cheese, coffee, tea, cola, and chocolate that contain caffeine; foods with yeast, such as pastry and fresh breads; foods that contain monosodium glutamate (MSG); and foods with nitrates for preservative such as pickled or fermented foods, nuts, artificial sweeteners, and smoked fish. Medications that should be considered triggers for migraine headache include cimetidine (Tagamet), estrogens, nitroglycerin (NTG), and nifedipine (Procardia). The factors that may trigger a migraine headache of which the client should be aware are anger, conflict, fatigue, light glare, missed meals, psychological stress, sleep problems, and pungent smells such as tobacco. The client should be instructed on the importance of discussing plans to take herbs with his or her health care provider, since herbs may cause drug-to-herbal interactions and trigger a migraine.

References

Broyles, B. E. (2005). *Medical-Surgical Nursing Clinical Companion*. Durham, NC: Carolina Academic Press.

Corbet, J. V. (2004). *Laboratory Tests and Diagnostic Procedures with Nursing Diagnoses* (6th ed.). Upper Saddle River, NJ: Prentice Hall.

Frisch, N. C. and Frisch, L. E. (2006). *Psychiatric Mental Health Nursing* (3rd ed.). Clifton Park, NY: Thomson Delmar Learning.

Gahart, B. L. and Nazareno, A. R. (2005). *2005 Intravenous Medications*. St. Louis: Elsevier Mosby.

Guyton, A. C. and Hall, J. E. (2006). Textbook of Medical Physiology (11th ed.). Philadelphia: W. B. Saunders.

Huether, S. E. and McCance, K. L. (2004). Understanding Pathophysiology (3rd ed.). St. Louis: Mosby.

Ignatavicius, D. D. and Workman, M. L. (2006). *Medical-Surgical Nursing across the Health Care Continuum* (5th ed.). Philadelphia: W. B. Saunders.

Kozier, B., Erb, G., Berman, A., and Snyder, S. (2004). *Fundamentals of Nursing: Concepts, Process, and Practice* (7th ed.). Upper Saddle River, NJ: Prentice Hall.

Smeltzer, C. S. and Bare, B. G. (2004). *Textbook of Medical-Surgical Nursing* (10th ed.). Philadelphia: Lippincott Williams & Wilkins.

Spratto, G. R. and Woods, A. L. (2005). *2005 Edition: PDR Nurse's Drug Handbook*. Clifton Park, NY: Thomson Delmar Learning.

CASE STUDY 2

Brain Tumor (Noninfiltrating Astrocytoma of the Cerebrum)

GENDER

F

AGE

52

SETTING

- Hospital

ETHNICITY/CULTURE

- Black American

PREEXISTING CONDITION

COEXISTING CONDITION

LIFESTYLE

- Employed full time as an RN in a community clinic
- Uses hair dyes to color hair occasionally

COMMUNICATION

DISABILITY

SOCIOECONOMIC STATUS

- Middle

SPIRITUAL/RELIGIOUS

- Seventh Day Adventist

PHARMACOLOGIC

- Acetaminophen (Tylenol)
- Chemotherapy/radiation therapy
- Glucocorticoid

PSYCHOSOCIAL

- Anxiety

LEGAL

ETHICAL

ALTERNATIVE THERAPY

- Homeopathic treatment, Oximax™

PRIORITIZATION

- Decrease intracranial pressure
- Transfer to neurology unit

DELEGATION

- RN
- Client education

THE NERVOUS SYSTEM

Level of difficulty: High

Overview: This case will focus on anaplastic astrocytoma, which is a highly malignant brain tumor. Because the prognosis of astrocytoma is poor, nurses must be skilled and sensitive, and have excellent communication skills to provide quality care that will maintain the highest quality of life possible. Nurses must also have optimum understanding of the treatment regimens for clients with this type of tumor.

DIFFICULT

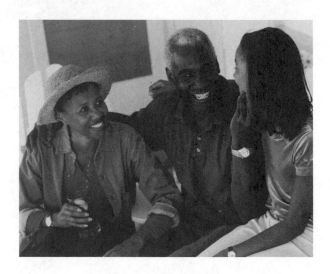

Client Profile

Mrs. S is a 52-year-old married woman and a registered nurse (RN) who is accompanied by her husband to the hospital emergency department (ED). On arrival, Mrs. S reports unusual ongoing headaches that go away for only brief periods after taking acetaminophen (Tylenol). Mr. S demonstrates concern for the complaints of unusual headaches. Mrs. S is 5'6" and weighs 128 pounds. (Her previous weight of two months ago was 140 pounds.)

Case Study

On initial interview, Mrs. S reports a history of nonsmall cell lung cancer and right lobectomy one year ago. She reports spending two weeks in Mexico for "homeopathic" treatment, including Oximax™ herbal supplement. Mrs. S reports that upon returning to the United States, she had a "good sense" of well-being. She also informs the admitting nurse that she is able to visit with her friends and remains involved with her daily chores, while returning to work part time. She reports enjoying changes in her hair color, which she occasionally gets at the beauty parlor. Mrs. S also reports that for the past month she has been unable to concentrate for long periods of time. The headaches continue and are more frequent and worse in the mornings, with two episodes of petit mal seizures occurring at different times after the onset of the headaches. The admitting health care provider did a thorough history and physical examination, focusing on the manner and time frame in which Mrs. S says the symptoms evolved.

After the examination, Mrs. S is transferred to the neurology unit. Her vital signs on arrival to the unit are:

Blood pressure: 130/78
Pulse: 78
Respirations: 20
Temperature: 98.8° F

She reports that the headaches have now subsided. The client requests that her husband remain with her and that he be present when the diagnosis is explained. The request is granted, and Mr. and Mrs. S are instructed to return to the hospital's outpatient clinic in one week to discuss the findings of the diagnostic studies and for confirmation of the diagnosis. Her vital signs are repeated:

Blood pressure: 130/78
Pulse: 76
Respirations: 16
Temperature: 98.8° F

She denies complaints of headaches. The following diagnostic and laboratory studies are ordered: magnetic resonance imaging (MRI), chest X-ray and plain skull radiograph, serum Na, K+, Hct, Hgb, WBC count, and PLT. They are scheduled and completed before Mrs. S leaves the hospital. The results of the diagnostic tests and lab results are received. The MRI reveals a mildly noninfiltrating astrocytoma of the cerebrum. The chest X-ray and plain skull radiographs are negative for metastasis. Other results:

Sodium (Na): 134
Potassium (K+): 4
Hematocrit (Hct): 34%
Hemoglobin (Hgb): 16 g/dL
White blood cell (WBC) count: 8,000
Platelet count (PLT): 200,000

Mr. and Mrs. S return to the clinic one week later as instructed. The results of the tests are reviewed with them. They are allowed to ask questions, and after appropriate dialogue, a diagnosis of brain tumor is explained to them. Mrs. S is asked to sign a witnessed, informed consent for the insertion of an Ommaya reservoir. The plans for treatment are discussed with them by an interdisciplinary team that includes an oncologist, a medical doctor, a surgical doctor, and an RN. Mrs. S is given a prescription for Percocet (5 mg PO to be taken q6h PRN) for headache until she returns in the morning to start outpatient chemotherapeutic treatment. The overall plan of care as it relates to the brain tumor is to admit Mrs. S to the hospital for administration of the first dosages of prescribed chemotherapeutic drugs over two days, then have her return in six weeks for repeat dosages and evaluation of the drug's effectiveness.

Questions

1. Discuss the pathophysiology of brain tumors.

2. Discuss different types of brain tumors.

3. Discuss common clinical manifestations of brain tumors.

4. Discuss diagnostic studies used to confirm brain tumors.

5. Discuss common nursing diagnoses for brain tumors.

6. Discuss the purpose for the Ommaya reservoir.

7. What are the purposes for the prescribed orders?

8. What are the most common adverse reactions, drug-to-drug, drug-to-food/herbal interactions for the prescribed medications?

9. Discuss treatment options for tumor excision.

10. Discuss client education for brain tumor.

Questions and Suggested Answers

1. Discuss the pathophysiology of brain tumors. Primary brain tumors arise either from the brain or its supporting structures. Tumors metastasizing from other areas in the body are secondary tumors. They are classified as space-occupying lesions because they displace normal tissue or occupy normal tissue spaces. Brain tumors that are classified as astrocytoma can range from low-grade to moderate-grade malignancy, with the most common primary brain tumors originating in astrocytes (cells). These are called gliomas and account for 65% of primary brain tumors. When normal brain tissue is compressed, blood flow is altered and ischemia leading to necrosis may occur, destroying major functions. Cancers of the lung, breast, and kidney and malignant melanoma are the major sources of metastatic brain cancers. Studies have shown that lung cancer is one of the commonly occurring tumors to metastasize to the brain. The current brain tumor may be related to a recurrence of cancer cells that have been in remission within the lung but are now active, resulting in release of cancer cells either from a primary lung tumor or a metastatic site in the lung.

2. Discuss different types of brain tumors. The incidence of brain tumors appears to have increased, and studies have cited that this is due to more aggressive and accurate diagnosis rather than an actual rise in the incidence. Brain tumors may be classified into several groups such as those arising from the coverings of the brain (i.e., dural meningioma), those developing in or on the cranial nerves (i.e. acoustic neuroma), those originating within the brain tissue (i.e., gliomas), and metastatic lesions originating within brain tissue. *Malignant glioma* is the most common brain neoplasm, and astrocytomas are the most common type of glioma. Astrocytoma refers to a pituitary tumor of the brain that is composed of astrocytes and is characterized by slow growth, cyst formation, invasion of surrounding structures, and often development of a highly malignant glioblastoma within the tumor mass. The pituitary gland is a small gland located in the sella turcia, is attached to the hypothalamus, and is divided into two lobes. Because of the anatomical position, *pituitary adenomas* are tumors that cause symptoms as a result of pressure on adjacent structures or hormonal changes (hyperfunction or hypofunction of the pituitary). The effects of pituitary tumors on the optic nerves, optic chiasm, or optic tracts or on the hypothalamus results in headache, visual dysfunction, hypothalmic disorders (e.g., sleep, appetite, temperature, emotions), increased intracranial pressure (ICP), and enlargement and erosion of the sella turcia. *Angiomas* are found either in or on the surface of the brain and occur in the cerebellum in 83% of cases. Some persist throughout life without causing any problems. However, because the walls of the blood vessels in angiomas are thin, these clients are at risk for a cerebral vascular accident (stroke). *Acoustic neuromas* are tumors of the eighth cranial nerve, the cranial nerve responsible for hearing and balance. The client usually experiences loss of hearing, tinnitus, and episodes of vertigo and staggering gait. As the tumor enlarges, painful sensations of the face may occur on the same side as a result of the tumor's compression of the fifth cranial nerve. *Meningiomas* are common benign encapsulated tumors of arachnoid cells on the meninges. They are slow growing and occur most often in middle-aged adults, and more often in women. Manifestations depend on the area involved and are the result of compression rather than invasion of brain tissue.

3. **Discuss common clinical manifestations of brain tumors.** The clinical manifestations of brain tumors depend mainly on the location and size of the tumor, with wide ranges of possible clinical manifestations. Headache is a common problem, which may be localized or generalized and are most severe in the frontal or occipital region. Headaches are usually intermittent, increasing in duration, and may be intensified by a change in posture or straining. Tumor-related headaches tend to be worse at night and may awaken the client. Seizures are common and are often the first manifestation of an intracranial mass. Seizures may occur due to the tumor pressing on neurons, resulting in spontaneous firing that spreads to the entire brain, depolarizing the neurons of the brain, resulting in seizure activity. Nausea and vomiting can occur due to increased pressure on the medulla of the brain, where the vomiting center is found. These manifestations may be related to generalized swelling, cerebral edema, increasing headache, and stimulation of the chemo-emetic trigger zone (CETZ). The CETZ has numerous neural connections from areas within the cerebral hemispheres that transmit or synapse with the vomiting center in the medulla. If headache is present, there is involvement with the CETZ, resulting in nausea and vomiting.

4. Discuss diagnostic studies used to confirm brain tumors. The chest X-ray is routine to look at the thoracic area for signs of metastasis of the left lung, and the plain skull X-ray provides information of its integrity and the need for advanced tests. The magnetic resonance imaging (MRI) and positron emission test (PET) allow for detection of very small tumors and may provide more reliable diagnostic information. Computed tomography (CT) scans and brain scanning are used to diagnose the location of the lesion.

5. Discuss common nursing diagnoses for brain tumors.
- Impaired tissue perfusion (cerebral) R/T cerebral edema – The nurse will need to assess neurologic status and vital signs frequently because the cerebrum is sensitive to lack of oxygen related to cerebral edema altering tissue perfusion. The head of the bed needs to be elevated at 30 degrees to help facilitate venous drainage and reduce edema.
- Acute pain (headache) R/T cerebral edema and increased ICP – The nurse will change the client's position slowly since rapid change in position increases cerebral blood flow and pressure, which increases pain. Administering steroids as ordered reduces cerebral edema and the pain related to the cerebral edema.
- Anxiety R/T fear of changes in body image or life expectancy – The nurse will anticipate the needs of the client to decrease anxiety and feelings of loneliness and provide the client with quality time to express feelings to help develop problem-solving coping styles. Offer reassurance and reasonable choices to reestablish feelings of control.
- Self-care deficits R/T altered neuromuscular function secondary to cerebral edema – The nurse will anticipate the client's needs, provide appropriate care, and gradually encourage self-care in a safe environment for the client.

6. Discuss the purpose for the Ommaya reservoir. The Ommaya reservoir is to ensure a more uniform distribution of chemotherapy to the fluid surrounding the brain and spinal cord. A surgeon places the catheter under the scalp, and injections with anticancer drugs are inserted into the catheter and then distributed evenly. This method avoids the discomfort of injections into the spine.

The following are prescribed:
- Dexamethasone sodium phosphate (Decadrol) IV 4 mg q4h for 24 hours
- Carmustine (BiCNU) IV 150 mg/m^2 over two days
- Lomustine (CeeNU) IV 130 mg/m^3 as a single dose, repeat in six weeks
- Phenytoin (Dilantin) 1 g PO as loading dose, then 100 mg PO three times per day
- Ranitidine hydrochloride (Zantac) 150 mg PO two times per day
- Serum labs: Na, K+, Hct, Hgb, WBC, platelet count before discharge

Discharge orders:

- Codeine phosphate 15 mg PO q three to six hours as needed
- Return to hospital oncology unit in six weeks for lomustine therapy

7. What are the purposes for the prescribed orders? *Codeine phosphate* relieves the pain. *Codeine phosphate* works to produce analgesia and relieve the headache by binding to opiate receptors in the CNS, altering the perception of and response to painful stimuli. *Dexamethasone sodium phosphate* controls cerebral edema by suppressing inflammation and modification of the normal immune response. Cerebral edema is a common occurrence with a tumor of the brain. *Carmustine* inhibits the synthesis of DNA and RNA, preventing reproduction of cancer cells and preventing their spread. *Carmustine* has a broad spectrum of activity against neoplastic diseases. Its effectiveness is significant in that it has the ability to cross the blood-brain barrier due to its lipid solubility. The high solubility makes it readily penetrate the blood-brain barrier, and effectively inhibit the synthesis of both DNA and RNA of the cells in all phases of the cell cycle. *Lomustine* inhibits the synthesis of DNA and RNA of the cells. Its action is similar to *carmustine*. However, *lomustine* is given orally and has a slower response time to act on the cancer cells. Both lomustine and carmustine enhance the action of each other. *Phenytoin* prevents recurrent seizure activities. Phenytoin is effective in preventing recurrent seizures because it inhibits seizure activity by stabilizing the seizure threshold against hyperexcitability, which reduces the maximal activity of brainstem centers that are responsible for seizure activity. *Ranitidine* decreases gastric acid secretion that usually develops due to the stress of the diagnosis and hospitalization. If the gastric acid secretion is not decreased, the client could develop a stress ulcer (Curling's ulcer). Ranitidine is effective in decreasing gastric acid because it blocks H_2 receptors on parietal cells, which are the cells that secrete hydrochloric acid. The serum labs, Na, K+, Hct, Hgb, WBC, and PLT are monitored before and during chemotherapy treatment, because the drugs suppress bone marrow function. Depending on the amount of suppression, dose adjustment will be implemented.

8. What are the most common adverse reactions, drug-to-drug, drug-to-food/herbal interactions for the prescribed medications? The most common adverse reactions of *dexamethasone* are depression, euphoria, hypertension, anorexia, nausea, acne, decreased wound healing, eccyhmoses, fragility, hirsutism, petechiae, adrenal suppression, muscle wasting, osteoporosis, nasal irritation, edema, hyperglycemia, oral candidiasis, and cushingcoid appearance. Drug-to-drug interactions may occur with the simultaneous use of thiazide and loop diuretics, amphotericin B, piperacillin, or ticarcillin, which may increase the risk of hypokalemia. Hypokalemia

may increase the risk of digoxin toxicity. The simultaneous use of insulin or oral hypoglycemic agents, phenytoin, phenobarbital, and rifampin may increase metabolism and decrease effectiveness of dexamethasone. The simultaneous use of hormonal contraceptives may decrease metabolism. The simultaneous use of nonsteroidal anti-inflammatory agents (NSAIDs) increases the risk of adverse gastrointestinal effects, and chronic doses may suppress adrenal function, decrease antibody response, and increase risk for adverse reactions from live-virus vaccines. The simultaneous use with fluoroquinolones may increase risk of tendon rupture, and concurrent use with somatrem or somatropin may decrease their response. The simultaneous use of antacid decreases the absorption of dexamethasone and prednisone. The simultaneous use of ketaconazole, itraconazole, ritonavir, indinavir, saquinavir, and erythromycin increases blood levels and effects of dexamethasone. Concurrent use with salicylate and isoniazid decreases their levels and effectiveness, and if used concurrently with anticholinesterases may antagonize its effects in myasthenia gravis. Drug-to-food interaction is seen with the use of grapefruit juice, which would increase the levels and effects of methylprednisone. There are no clinically significant drug-to-herbal interactions established. The most common adverse reactions of *carmustine* are hepatoxicity, stomatitis, nausea, and vomiting. Drug-to-drug interactions may occur with the simultaneous use of antineoplastics, radiation therapy, or cimetidine, which may increase bone marrow suppression and significant neutropenia and thrombocytopenia. There are no clinically significant drug-to-food/herbal interactions established. The most common adverse reactions, drug-to-drug/ food/herbal interactions are similar to carmustine. The most common adverse reactions of *phenytoin* are ataxia, diplopia, nystagmus, hypotension, nausea, hypertrichosis, rashes, drowsiness, gingival hyperplasia, and Steven's-Johnson syndrome. Drug-to-drug interaction may occur with the simultaneous use of alcohol, amiodarone, chloramphenicol, isoniazid, influenzae vaccine, sulfonamides, fluoxetine, benzodiapizines, omeprazole, ticlopidine, itraconazole, ketoconazole, fluconazole, miconazole, estrogens, halothane, methylphenidate, phenothiazines, salicylates, tolbutamide, trazodone, felbamate, and cimetidine, which may increase phenytoin blood levels. Carbamazepine, reserpine, and chronic ingestion of alcohol may decrease phenytoin blood levels. Phenytoin may alter the effects of felbamate, corticosteroids, doxycycline, rifampin, quinidine, methadone, cyclosporine, and estrogens. The simultaneous use with dopamine may cause additive hypotension, and additive CNS depression may occur with the simultaneous use of other CNS depressants including alcohol, antihistamines, antidepressants, opioid analgesics, and sedative/hypnotics. Antacids may decrease absorption of orally administered phenytoin and may decrease the effectiveness of streptozocin or theophylline. Additive cardiac depression may occur with the simultaneous use of propranolol or lidocaine. The simultaneous use of calcium and sulcralfate decrease pheyntoin effects in clients stabilized on warfarin therapy. Drug-to-food interactions may occur with simultaneous use of folic acid, calcium, and vitamin D. Phenytoin may decrease the absorption, and gingko may decrease phenytoin's effectiveness. There are no clinically significant drug-to-herbal interactions established. The most common adverse reaction of *ranitidine Hcl* is confusion. Drug-to-drug interactions may occur with ketoconazole, delavirdine, itraconazole, and cefuroxime, benzodiazepines (especially chlordiazepoxide, diazepam, and midazolam), some beta blockers (labetalol, metoprolol, propranolol), caffeine, calciumchannel blockers, carbamazepine, chloroquine, lidocaine, metronidazole, moricizine, pentoxifylline, phenytoin, propafenone, quinidine, quinine, metformin, sulfonylureas, tracrine, theophylline, triamterene, tricyclic antidepressants, valproic acid, and warfarin may increase levels and toxic effects. The simultaneous use of succinylcholine, flecainide, procainamide, carmustine, and fluorouracil effects increase with the simultaneous use of cimetidine. There are no clinically significant drug-to-food/herbal interactions established. The most common adverse reactions of *codeine phosphate* are confusion, sedation, hypotension, dizziness, nausea, vomiting, lightheadedness, pruritus, and constipation. Drug-to-drug interaction is seen with the simultaneous use of other CNS depressant drugs (i.e., alcohol, antidepressants, antihistamines, and sedative/hypnotics) may result in additive CNS depression. The simultaneous use of partial antagonists (buprenorphine, butorphanol, nalbuphine, or pentazocine) may precipitate opioid withdrawal in physically dependent clients. The simultaneous use with pentazocine may decrease analgesia. Drug-to-food/herbal interactions may occur with the simultaneous use of St. John's Wort, kava, valerian, skullcap, chamomile, or hops, which may increase CNS depressants.

9. Discuss treatment options for tumor excision. The neurosurgeon may choose to do *embolization* of the tumor in conjunction with surgery. Embolization interrupts the arterial blood flow to tumors, resulting in shrinking and destruction of the tumor. *Laser surgery* may be used to destroy tumor tissue. The heat from the laser destroys the tumor without causing adjacent edema or damage. *Polymer wafer implants (chemotherapeutic wafers)* are placed in the tumor bed, and carmustine is currently being used to eradicate some tumors.

10. Discuss client teaching for brain tumor. Because noninfiltrating astrocytoma can progress to anaplastic astrocytoma, follow-up care is warranted with CT scan or MRI to monitor effectiveness of prior treatments or progression of the tumor. Oral codeine phosphate can cause confusion, sedation, hypotension, constipation, nausea, and vomiting. Client should maintain safety measures at all times and avoid operating a vehicle if feeling drowsy.

Include foods high in roughage in diet and increase fluids to decrease constipation. If feeling nauseated, client should lie down because nausea is aggravated by ambulation. Notify primary health care provider if the symptom persists. Do not take alcohol or other CNS depressants unless approved by health care provider.

References

Black, J. M. and Hawks, J. H (2005). *Medical-Surgical Nursing: Clinical Management for Positive Outcomes*. Philadelphia: W. B. Saunders.

Broyles, B. E. (2005). *Medical-Surgical Nursing Clinical Companion*. Durham, NC: Carolina Academic Press.

Gahart, B. L. and Nazareno, A. R. (2005). *2005 Intravenous Medications*. St. Louis: Mosby.

Huether, S. E. and McCance, K. L. (2004). *Understanding Pathophysiology* (3rd ed.). St. Louis: Mosby.

Ignatavicius, D. D. and Workman, M. L. (2006). *Medical-Surgical Nursing across the Health Care Continuum* (5th ed.). Philadelphia: W. B. Saunders.

Spratto, G. R. and Woods, A. L. (2005). *2005 Edition: PDR Nurse's Drug Handbook*. Clifton Park, NY: Thomson Delmar Learning.

Parkinson's Disease

GENDER

M

AGE

70

SETTING

- Health care provider's office

ETHNICITY/CULTURE

- White American

PREEXISTING CONDITIONS

COEXISTING CONDITIONS

LIFESTYLE

- Retired postal employee

COMMUNICATION

DISABILITY

- Yes

SOCIOECONOMIC STATUS

- Middle

SPIRITUAL/RELIGIOUS

- Presbyterian

PHARMACOLOGIC

- Entacapone (Comtan)
- Carbidopa/levodopa (Sinemet)
- Amantadine HcL (Symmetrel)

PSYCHOSOCIAL

- Anxiety
- Fear
- Depression

LEGAL

- Clients with PD should have optimum care regardless of the financial resources and health insurance they may have.

ETHICAL

- Should federal funding be available for all persons with PD?

ALTERNATIVE THERAPY

- Exercise
- Walking
- Gingko biloba

PRIORITIZATION

- Prevent aspiration
- Maintain safety

DELEGATION

- RN
- Client education

M O D E R A T E

THE NERVOUS SYSTEM

Level of difficulty: Moderate

Overview: This case involves thorough assessment of the client's condition including drugs or herbals he is currently taking. It also involves gathering of past medical history to assist in determining the symptomatic causes of the disease process. The nurse must be skilled at identifying critical symptoms and implementing short- and long-term goals for clinical management of presenting symptoms. The nurse must also be aware of the pharmacologic agents that are effective in slowing the disease progression.

Client Profile

Mr. A is a 70-year-old married man who is accompanied by his 65-year-old wife to the family's primary health care provider, who is a part of a medical group, for his annual physical examination. Mrs. A's primary report during the history is that she has observed minor changes in Mr. A for several months but related them to him getting older. Mrs. A reports that there is a noted progression of unusual looks on his face; resting tremors of the extremities; a slow and shuffling gait and difficulty stopping quickly, which she says is new; and rigidity and abnormally slow movements, which causes him to take much longer to complete most basic activities such as getting dressed and feeding himself. She also reports "pill-rolling" movements and difficulty chewing and swallowing at mealtimes.

Case Study

Mr. A's vital signs are:

Blood pressure: 100/70
Pulse: 72 and regular
Respirations: 14
Temperature: 98.6° F

The neurologist completes the history and physical examination. The subjective data is reviewed with Mr. A's spouse, and quality time is spent discussing the findings. A diagnosis of Parkinson's disease (PD) is confirmed, and the multidisciplinary team, including the neurologist, medical doctor, registered dietitian, registered nurse (RN), nurse practitioner, rehabilitation staff, speech-language pathologist, social worker, and case manager, discuss the case further. A plan of care for Mr. A. is made. The final decision on placement is made by Mr. A and his wife. Both of them agree that he will return to his home and continue with reevaluation monthly or more frequently, as needed. The case manager, social worker, registered dietitian, and rehabilitation staff initiate home-care services.

Questions

1. Discuss the pathophysiology of Parkinson's disease (PD).

2. Discuss common clinical manifestations of PD.

3. Discuss other manifestations of PD.

4. Discuss assessment and diagnostic findings of PD.

5. Discuss the medical and nursing management of PD.

6. Discuss the "on-off" response that occurs with PD.

7. What are the purposes for the prescribed orders?

Questions (continued)

8. What are the most common adverse reactions, drug-to-drug, drug-to-food/herbal interactions of the prescribed medications?

9. Discuss stereotactic procedures used with PD.

10. Discuss client education for PD.

Questions and Suggested Answers

1. Discuss the pathophysiology of Parkinson's disease (PD). Parkinson's disease (PD) is a neurologic disorder of older adults. It is a chronic, progressive disease that results from loss of the neurotransmitter dopamine in a group of brain structures that control movement. When PD occurs, degenerative changes are found in an area of the brain known as the substantia nigra, which produces dopamine, a chemical substance that enables people to move normally and smoothly. The cause of nigral cell degeneration is not known, but once cell loss reaches 80%, manifestations appear. However, new evidence has found that the disease not only affects movement due to dopamine loss from the brain, but also involves the autonomic nervous system, with norepinephrine being lost in the nervous system of the heart. This loss results in orthostatic hypotension, which is frequently seen in the client with PD.

2. Discuss common clinical manifestations of PD. *Tremor* that is slow and unilateral, and resting tremor that is presenting in 70% of clients at the time of diagnosis. The resting tremors disappear with purposeful movements but are evident as the extremities maintain a motionless position, and they increase with walking. *Muscle rigidity* is evident by resistance to passive limb movement. Passive movement of an extremity may cause it to move in jerky increments referred to as *"cogwheeling."* *Stiffness* of the neck, trunk, and shoulders is common, and early in the disease, the client may complain of shoulder pain. *Bradykinesia*, in which clients take longer to complete most activities and have difficulty initiating movement, such as rising from a sitting position or turning in bed, is one of the most common features of PD. *Hypokinesia* (abnormally diminished movements) is common and may appear after the tremor. There may be the *"freezing phenomenon,"* which is a transient inability to perform active movement and is thought to be an extreme form of bradykinesia. *Micrographia* (shrinking, slowing handwriting) is evident as dexterity declines. *Mask-like faces* without expression and decreased frequency of blinking. *Speech* is soft, slurred, low pitched, and less audible. Clients often develop *dysphagia*, begin to drool, and are at risk for choking and aspiration. There are postural and gait problems with loss of postural reflexes. Therefore, the client stands with

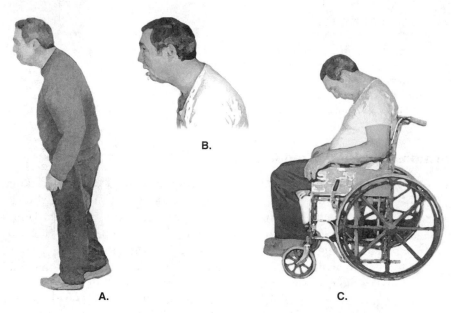

The shuffling gate and early postural change of Parkinson's disease (A and B). Drooling, head held forward, and inability to stand are common in the advanced stages of the disease (C).

head bent forward and walks with a ***propulsive gait***. This posture is caused by the forward flexion of the neck, hips, knees, and elbows. The client tries to walk faster, trying to move the feet forward under the body's center of gravity (***shuffling gait***). There is difficulty in pivoting, and loss of balance (either forward or backward) places the client at risk for falls.

3. Discuss other manifestations of PD. PD affects the basal ganglia (four masses or substances of gray matter located deep in the cerebral hemisphere). The functions of the basal ganglia are complex and include some of the subconscious aspects of voluntary movement such as accessory movements and inhibiting tremor. Therefore, the effects result in autonomic symptoms that include excessive and uncontrolled sweating, orthostatic hypotension, gastric and urinary retention, and constipation. Sleep disorders and depression are also common, but it has not been established if the depression is due to biochemical abnormality. A number of psychiatric manifestations occur, such as personality changes, psychosis, dementia, and acute confusion.

4. Discuss assessment and diagnostic findings of PD. Laboratory tests and imaging studies are not helpful in the diagnosis of PD, although position emission tomography (PET) scanning has been used in the evaluation of levodopa uptake and conversion to dopamine in the corpus striatum (a structure in the cerebral hemispheres consisting of two basal ganglia).

Currently, the disease is diagnosed clinically from the client's history and the presence of two of the three cardinal manifestations: tremor, muscle rigidity, and bradykinesia. The medical history, presenting symptoms, neurologic examination, and response to pharmacologic management are carefully evaluated when making the diagnosis.

5. Discuss the medical and nursing management of PD. Because there are no medical or surgical approaches that prevent disease progression, treatment is directed at controlling symptoms and maintaining the client's functional independence. Pharmacologic management is currently the mainstay of treatment, although advances in research have led to increased interest in surgical interventions. In 2003, the Food and Drug Administration (FDA) approved Stalevo to help with the improvement of Parkinson's symptoms. Stalevo works by extending the benefits of levodopa and, in doing so, improves the control of Parkinson's symptoms. Studies cite that Stalevo begins working immediately in some clients, but with others, it may take a few days to notice improvement.

6. Discuss the "on-off" response that occurs with PD. An "on/off" response refers to rapid fluctuation of clinical manifestations that may occur when the client is mobile and active ("on") one moment and akinetic and rigid ("off") the next. This transmission may happen quickly, within one or two minutes. Initially, the "off" periods tend to occur three or four hours after a dose of anti-Parkinson's medication. Later the transition may happen at any time and be unrelated to medication ingestion. It is believed that "off" periods are due to dopamine deficit.

The following are prescribed:

- Entacapone (Comtan) 200 mg PO three times per day with Sinemet
- Carbidopa/levodopa (Sinemet) 10 mg carbidopa/100 mg levodopa PO three times per day
- Amantadine HcL (Symmetrel) 100 mg PO daily

7. What are the purposes for the prescribed orders? *Entacapone* is a selective and reversible catechol-O-methyltransferase inhibitor and an anti-Parkinson's drug that reduces the symptoms of PD by blocking the breakdown of levodopa in the body so more can travel to the brain and convert to dopamine. *Carbidopa/levodopa* also is classified as an anti-Parkinson's agent that helps to decrease tremors, rigidity, and bradykinesia, thereby aiding in the restoration of dopamine levels in extrapyramidal centers that are depleted of dopamine in persons with PD. *Carbidopa/levodopa* accomplishes its action because levodopa is converted in the brain into dopamine, and the dopamine then restores the normal balance between inhibition and excitation in the brain. *Amantadine HcL* is an anti-Parkinson's agent. The mechanism of amantadine HcL action in PD is not clearly understood, but it may be related to release of dopamine and other catecholamines from neuronal storage sites, and improve symptoms.

8. **What are the most common adverse reactions, drug-to-drug, drug-to-food/herbal interactions for the prescribed medications?** The most common adverse reactions of *entacapone* are dyskinesia, hyperkinesia, hypokinesia, dizziness, anxiety, somnolence, agitation, fatigue, nausea, diarrhea, and urine discoloration. Drug-to-drug interactions may occur with the simultaneous use of *entacapone* and bitolterol, dobutamine, dopamine, epinephrine, isoetharine, isoproterenol, methyldopa, and norepinephrine may increase heart rates and possibly cause arrythmias and excessive changes in blood pressure. Ampicillin, chloramphenicol, erythromycin, probenecid, and rifampin decrease the biliary excretion of *entacapone*. If used concurrently with monoamine oxidase (MAO) inhibitors, a significant increase in the levels of catecholamines may occur. No clinically significant drug-to-food/herbal interactions have been established. The most common adverse reaction of *carbidopa/levodopa* are kinesias, choreiform, and involuntary movements, orthostatic hypotension, blepharospasm, anorexia, nausea, and vomiting. Clients abruptly withdrawn from levodopa may experience neuroleptic malignant-like syndrome including muscular rigidity, hyperthermia, increased serum phosphokinase, and alterations in mental status (Spratto and Woods, 185). With *carbidopa/levodopa* drug-to-drug interactions may occur with the simultaneous use of MAO inhibitors, which may precipitate hypertensive crisis; tricyclic antidepressants may cause postural hypotension; haloperidol may antagonize the therapeutic effects of levodopa; pyridoxine may reverse the effects of carbidopa/levodopa; methyldopa may increase toxic central nervous system (CNS) effects. Drug-to-food interaction results in the decrease in the rate and extent of carbidopa/levodopa absorption. Drug-to-herbal interaction is seen with the simultaneous use of kava-kava, which may worsen Parkinsonian symptoms. Common adverse reactions of *amantadine HcL* are confusion, lightheadedness, anxiety, nausea, and constipation. Drug-to-drug interactions may also occur with the simultaneous use of anticholinergics and levodopa, as these agents potentiate the effects of *amantadine*. If used with CNS depressants, the CNS and psychic effects of *amantadine* may be increased. Hydrochlorothiazide/triamterene combination, trimethoprim/sulfamethoxazole, and quinidine decrease renal clearance of *amantadine* and increase the plasma levels. No clinically significant drug-to-food interactions have been established, however, herbal interactions have been documented. Belladonna leaf/root, henbane leaf, Pheasant's eye herb, and scopolia root increase the effects of *amantadine*.

9. **Discuss stereotactic procedures used with PD.** The use of transplanted fetal dopamine cells (not yet effective for more than a few months). Destroying part of the feedback circuitry in the basal ganglia to the motor cortex. Deep brain stimulation (DBS) reduces the need for levodopa and related

drugs. DBS is now approved by the U.S. Food and Drug Administration and is widely used as a treatment of PD. Cell replacement through transplantation is an emerging approach for repairing the damage PD causes in the brain.

10. Discuss client education for PD. Written instructions should be given to the client, spouse, and significant others, and the instructions should be clarified before discharge. The client and significant others should be taught about home safety. Loose carpeting should be removed. Grab bars should be placed in the bathroom. An elevated toilet seat should be installed. If tremor is severe, clients should not carry hot foods. The client should be taught to rise slowly from a sitting or lying position to avoid feelings of dizziness. Prescribed medications must be taken on schedule with meals, and the client should avoid missing a dose. Entacapone may cause the urine to be brownish-orange. This is an expected response of the drug, therefore do not stop taking the drug. If the client begins to hallucinate or have persistent nausea or diarrhea, report these symptoms to the health care provider. However, these are often due to the present dose of the drug, which can be adjusted. The client must rinse the mouth out frequently with sips of water to prevent drying of the mouth. Significant others should report all mental status changes to the health care provider promptly. Shortness of breath, edema of the lower extremities, and unusual weight gain should be reported. The health care provider should be immediately made aware of signs of unusual slowness of movement or speech, rigidity, and tremors, as they indicate worsening of the condition that needs emergency care. Information concerning referrals, needs to be discussed, including the names and contact numbers of the persons involved.

References

Broyles, B. E. (2005). *Medical-Surgical Nursing Clinical Companion*. Durham, NC: Carolina Academic Press.

Corbet, J. V. (2004). *Laboratory Tests and Diagnostic Procedures with Nursing Diagnoses* (6th ed.). Upper Saddle River, NJ: Prentice Hall.

Deglin, J. H. and Vallerand, A. H. (2005). *Davis's Drug Guide for Nurses* (9th ed.). Philadelphia: F. A. Davis.

"FDA Approves Stavelo™ for Treatment of Parkinson's Disease." Available at www.pharma.us.novartis.com (accessed December 2005).

Gahart, B. L. and Nazareno, A. R. (2005). *2005 Intravenous Medications*. St. Louis: Elsevier Mosby.

Huether, S. E. and McCance, K. L. (2004). *Understanding Pathophysiology* (3rd ed.). St. Louis: Mosby.

Ignatavicius, D. D. and Workman, M. L. (2006). *Medical-Surgical Nursing across the Health Care Continuum* (5th ed.). Philadelphia: W. B. Saunders.

"Parkinson's Disease: Challenges, Progress, and Promise." Available at www.ninds.nih.gov (accessed July 2005).

Spratto, G. R. and Woods, A. L. (2005). *2005. Edition: PDR Nurse's Drug Handbook*. Clifton Park, NY: Thomson Delmar Learning.

PART FIVE

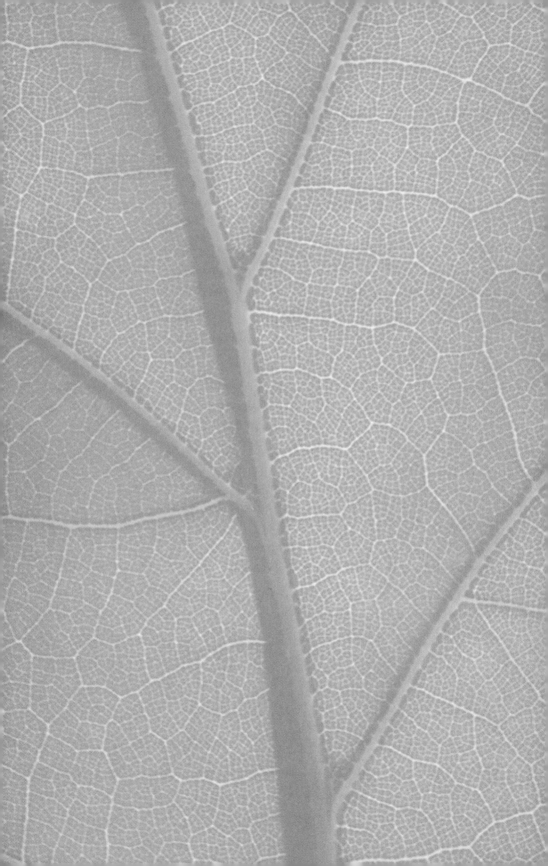

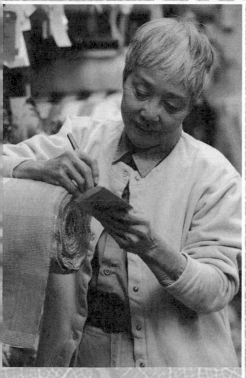

The Endocrine System

Diabetes Mellitus (Noninsulin Diabetes Mellitus Type 2)

E A S Y

GENDER

F

AGE

50

SETTING

- Health care provider's office

ETHNICITY/CULTURE

- Black American

PREEXISTING CONDITIONS

- Hypertension
- Obesity
- HDL less than 35 mg/dl
- Triglyceride levels >250

COEXISTING CONDITIONS

LIFESTYLE

- Elementary school teacher

COMMUNICATION

DISABILITY

SOCIOECONOMIC STATUS

- Middle

SPIRITUAL/RELIGIOUS

- Methodist

PHARMACOLOGIC

- Nateglinide (Starlix)

PSYCHOSOCIAL

- Concern

LEGAL

ETHICAL

ALTERNATIVE THERAPY

- Prayer
- Herbal teas

PRIORITIZATION

- Stabilize glucose levels
- Prevent complications

DELEGATION

- RN
- Client education

THE ENDOCRINE SYSTEM

Level of difficulty: Easy

Overview: This case involves a thorough assessment of the client's condition, including family history of diabetes, history of cigarette smoking, exercise, dietary habits, and current medications and herbals the client is currently taking. The nurse must be knowledgeable about the incidence, prevalence, and long-term complications of untreated diabetes mellitus. The nurse must first determine what the client understands about diabetes mellitus, then reinforce and clarify necessary components of the disease to enhance compliance with prescribe regimen.

Client Profile

Ms. E is a 50-year-old woman who is seen in her primary health care provider's office as an "add-on" for the day's schedule. Ms. E is 5'4" and weighs 190 pounds. Her past medical history includes hypertension and recent complaints of stiffness and discomfort of the upper extremities, especially on awakening.

Case Study

Ms. E denies smoking or alcohol intake of any kind. Her reason for seeking medical attention by her primary health care provider is related to a noted increase in urination during the day, waking from sleep in the night to urinate, and occasional blurred vision. Her vital signs are done by the office nurse and are:

Blood pressure: 138/80
Pulse: 78 and regular
Respirations: 14
Temperature: 98.4° F

An electrocardiogram (EKG) is done, Ms. E's height and weight is remeasured, and a nurse technician accompanies the client to the health care provider's office. After discussion on the reasons for the visit, a history and physical exam are done, the EKG results discussed, and the following laboratory orders are prescribed: fasting blood glucose, glycosylated hemoglobin assays (HbA$_{1c}$). Ms. E is given instructions on preparation for these tests and is referred to a laboratory agency to have the tests done. She is given an appointment to return to the health care provider's office in two weeks. A tentative diagnosis of diabetes mellitus type 2 is made, and Ms. E is given educational material on diabetes and instructed by the office nurse to increase daily exercise and decrease fat and caloric intake as per a dietary chart included in the educational material on diabetes. The office nurse demonstrates the use of a glucose-monitoring machine, and Ms. E gives return demonstration in preparation for using the machine at home. A glucometer machine and supplies are given to her to initiate monitoring her blood glucose twice per day for two weeks (in the morning on awaking and after her evening meal, preferably no later than 6 PM). Ms. E is to keep a record of the glucose levels and bring the record with her at the follow-up visit.

Ms. E returns to the health care provider's office in two weeks as scheduled, and the following lab results were reviewed with her:

Fasting blood glucose: 138 mg/dl
Glycosylated hemoglobin assays (HbA$_{1c}$): 6.5%

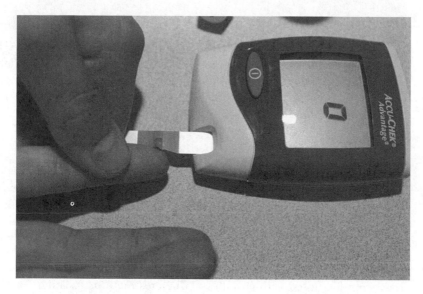

Glucose monitor.

Self-monitoring blood glucose (SMBG): within range of 134 mg/dL to 154 mg/dL

The health care provider reviews the results of the tests and Ms. E's SMBG reports then confirms a diagnosis of noninsulin dependent diabetes mellitus based on the reports and subjective data.

Questions

1. Discuss the incidence, prevalence, and pathophysiology of type 2 diabetes mellitus.

2. Discuss the major risk factors of type 2 diabetes mellitus.

3. Discuss the criteria for the diagnosis of type 2 diabetes mellitus.

4. Discuss special considerations for type 2 diabetes mellitus.

5. Discuss common nursing diagnoses of type 2 diabetes mellitus.

6. Discuss other prescribed oral agents for clients with type 2 diabetes who are not controlled by dietary regimen.

7. Discuss considerations for older adults who take antidiabetic oral agents.

8. What are the purposes for the prescribed orders?

9. What are the most common adverse reactions, drug-to-drug, and drug-to-food/herbal interactions for the prescribed medication?

10. If Ms. E develops Hyperglycemic Hyperosmolar Nonketotic Syndrome (HHNS), what are the key features for which the nurse would monitor?

11. Discuss client education for type 2 diabetes mellitus.

Questions and Suggested Answers

1. Discuss the incidence, prevalence, and pathophysiology of type 2 diabetes mellitus. About 90% of persons with diabetes have type 2 diabetes. Diagnosed diabetes is most common among middle-aged and older adults, affecting about 6% of people 45–64 years of age and 11% of those over 65 years of age. About 10% of clients diagnosed with diabetes are older than 70 years of age. After 40 years of age, new-onset diabetes is usually type 2. The prevalence of diabetes is similar for men and women. Although type 2 diabetes is a disease of middle-aged and older adults, recent studies show an increase of the disorder in childhood and adolescence as a result of obesity.

2. Discuss the major risk factors of type 2 diabetes mellitus. The client may have a first-degree relative with diabetes; is habitually physically inactive; is a member of a high-risk ethnic population (e.g., African American, Hispanic American, Native American/American Indian, Asian American, or Pacific Islander); delivered a baby weighing more than nine pounds or has been diagnosed with gestational diabetes mellitus (GDM); has history of hypertension (greater than 140/90 mm Hg), high-density lipoprotein cholesterol (HDL) less than 35 mg/dL, polycystic ovary syndrome, IFG or IGT on previous testing, and/or a history of vascular disease.

3. Discuss the criteria for the diagnosis of type 2 diabetes mellitus. Symptoms of diabetes plus casual blood glucose concentration greater than 200 mg/dL *or* fasting plasma glucose greater than 126 mg/dL *or* two-hour plasma glucose greater than 200 mg/dL during an oral glucose tolerance test. *Note: Each test must be confirmed on a subsequent day under similar circumstances.*

4. Discuss special considerations for type 2 diabetes mellitus. Many clients with type 2 diabetes are overweight and insulin resistant. Diet therapy stresses lifestyle changes that reduce calories eaten and increase calories expended through physical activity. Many clients with diabetes also have abnormal blood fat levels (metabolic syndrome) and hypertension, making reductions of saturated fat, cholesterol, and sodium desirable. A moderate caloric restriction (250–500 calories less than average daily intake) and an increase in physical activity improve diabetic control and weight control. Decreases of more than 10% of body weight can result in significant improvement in glycosylated hemoglobin. Decreasing intake of cholesterol-raising fatty acids helps reduce the risk of cardiovascular disease.

5. Discuss common nursing diagnoses for clients with type 2 diabetes.
- Health Maintenance, Altered R/T lack of knowledge about diabetes mellitus – The nurse or diabetes educator will relate the basic pathophysiologic mechanism of diabetes mellitus, will explain the purpose for exercise and diet in the treatment plan, and will list the clinical manifestations of acute and chronic complications.

- Health Maintenance, Altered R/T blood glucose and urine ketone testing – All newly diagnosed diabetes mellitus clients require teaching about blood glucose monitoring. In addition to demonstrating the techniques of blood glucose self-monitoring, the nurse should discuss the normal glucose range, individualized goals for good control, when to test, how to record test results. The nurse can consult a diabetic educator for assistance in helping the client choose the right glucometer.
- Health Maintenance, Altered R/T lack of knowledge about dietary management of diabetes – The nurse will consult with the registered dietitian (preferably a certified diabetes educator) for the initial evaluation and teaching any client with a new diagnosis of diabetes mellitus. Each client should receive an individualized meal plan based on ethnic, religious, and cultural background; eating, cooking, and work habits; and food preferences.
- Health Maintenance, Altered R/T exercise and foot care – The client will be taught the different types of exercises and that he or she should consult with the health care provider about the type of exercise the client should participate in. Exercise of short duration and of low to moderate intensity involves walking a half-mile or leisurely bicycling for less than 30 minutes. Exercise should gradually increase, depending on the client's tolerance. The client will be taught the importance of daily foot care. The client will be instructed to inspect feet using a mirror if necessary to see the bottom of the foot, including inspection for cracks between toes. Daily washing of feet in warm water with soap, and drying feet thoroughly. Applying lotion to entirety of feet, except between the web of the toes. Wear proper fitting shoes, and consult with a certified podiatrist for regular toenail care.

6. Discuss other prescribed oral agents for clients with type 2 diabetes who are not controlled by dietary regimen. *Sulfonylurea agents* are used only for clients with some remaining pancreatic beta-cell function. These drugs stimulate insulin secretion and enhance the number or sensitivity of cell receptor sites for interaction with insulin. *Hypoglycemia* is the most serious complication of sulfonylurea therapy. *Meglitinide Analogs* has a rapid onset with limited duration of action and is taken before meals. *Hypoglycemia* is one of its adverse effects. *Biguanides* include the drug metformin (Glucophage), which lowers glucose by decreasing liver glucose release and decreasing cellular insulin resistance. It does not stimulate insulin release. When given alone it does not cause hypoglycemia. It should not be used in conditions that decrease drug clearance such as renal insufficiency, liver disease, alcoholism, severe congestive heart failure, or to clients older than 80 years of age. *Alpha-Glucosidase inhibitors* include the drug miglitol

(Glyset), which should be taken three times daily with the first bite of each main meal. *Alpha-Glucosidase inhibitors* do not cause hypoglycemia unless given with sulfonylureas or insulin. *Thiazolidinediones* include the drug rosiglitazone (Avandia). These drugs are known as insulin sensitizers because they improve sensitivity to insulin in muscle and fat tissue and inhibit gluconeogenesis. Weight gain is a common side effect of these drugs, and there is a potential for liver damage. *Combination drugs*, such as glucovance, combines glyburide with metformin, resulting in maintaining desired blood glucose control.

7. Discuss considerations for older adults who take antidiabetic oral agents. Older clients who take antidiabetic drugs are at increased risk for hypoglycemia. Age-related changes in liver and kidney function slow metabolism of these drugs, predisposing the client to prolonged and recurrent hypoglycemia. Older clients may have a delayed release of epinephrine in response to falling blood glucose levels and are less likely to notice and act on hypoglycemic symptoms. Physical symptoms such as confusion may make older clients unable to correct hypoglycemia. When possible, an antidiabetic drug with low hypoglycemia potential is selected for older clients. The highest risk for severe or fatal hypoglycemia is among older adults taking glyburide.

The following are prescribed:

- Nateglinide (Starlix) 60 mg PO three times per day
- 2,000-calorie weight reduction diet
- Daily regular exercise

8. What are the purposes for the prescribed orders? *Nateglinide* lowers blood glucose by triggering insulin secretion via interaction with the adenosine triphosphate (ATP)-sensitive potassium channel on pancreatic beta cells. Because the drug is rapidly absorbed, it stimulates insulin secretion within 20 minutes of ingestion. The *2,000-calorie weight reduction diet* helps keep blood glucose and glycosylated hemoglobin levels as near normal as possible. The *daily regular exercise* helps regulate blood glucose levels and improves diabetic control by increasing insulin sensitivity, improves cell uptake of glucose, and promotes weight loss. Physical exercise reduces the insulin requirement and improves glucose tolerance. Regular exercise also decreases the risk for cardiovascular diseases, which are seen in chronic diabetes mellitus.

9. What are the most common adverse drug reactions, drug-to-drug, drug-to-food/herbal interactions for the prescribed medication? There are no common adverse reactions of *nateglinide.* Drug-to-drug interactions may occur with the simultaneous use of beta blockers, which may mask hypoglycemia. The simultaneous use of alcohol, other antidiabetics, nonsteroidal anti-inflammatory agents (NSAIDs), monoamine oxidase (MAO)

inhibitors, nonselective beta blockers may increase the risk of hypoglycemia. The simultaneous use with thiazide diuretics, corticosteroids, thyroid supplements, or adrenergic agents may decrease hypoglycemia effects. Drug-to-food interactions may occur if given prior to liquid meals. Drug-to-herbal interactions may occur with the simultaneous use of garlic and ginseng, which may potentiate hypoglycemic effects.

10. If Ms. E develops Hyperglycemic Hyperosmolar Nonketotic Syndrome (HHNS), what are the key features for which the nurse would monitor? Serum glucose greater than 800 mg/dL; osmolarity greater than 350 mOsm/L; negative serum ketones; serum pH greater than 7.4; serum HCO_3 greater than 20 mEq/L; normal or low serum sodium; normal or low serum potassium; elevated blood urea nitrogen (BUN); elevated creatinine; and negative urine ketones.

11. Discuss client education for type 2 diabetes mellitus. Clients should be aware that antidiabetic drugs are not a substitute for dietary modification and exercise. The nurse needs to be sure the client knows how to self-monitor blood glucose and how often she should do so. The client needs reinforcement concerning dietary instructions about the ADA exchange list (from the American Diabetes Association) and how to modify her carbohydrate intake. The client should be taught the signs and symptoms of hyperglycemia and hypoglycemia, and how to properly do daily foot care. The client needs medication instructions including the name of the drug, the dosage, the frequency of administration, and any adverse effects. The clients needs to be taught the importance of routine medical follow-up care. The client needs to consult with their primary health care provider or pharmacist before using over-the-counter medications.

References

Broyles, B. E. (2005). *Medical-Surgical Nursing Clinical Companion*. Durham, NC: Carolina Academic Press.

Corbet, J. V. (2004). *Laboratory Tests and Diagnostic Procedures with Nursing Diagnoses*. (6th ed.). Upper Saddle River, NJ: Prentice Hall.

Diabetes Mellitus. Various articles. Available at www.niddk.nih.gov.

Gahart, B. L. and Nazareno, A. R. (2005). *2005 Intravenous Medications*. St. Louis: Elsevier Mosby.

Huether, S. E. and McCance, K. L. (2004). *Understanding Pathophysiology* (3rd ed.). St. Louis: Mosby.

Ignatavicius, D. D. and Workman, M. L. (2006). *Medical-Surgical Nursing across the Health Care Continuum* (5th ed.). Philadelphia: W. B. Saunders.

Spratto, G. R. and Woods, A. L. (2005). *2005 Edition: PDR Nurse's Drug Handbook*. Clifton Park, NY: Thomson Delmar Learning.

Hypoparathyroidism

GENDER

F

AGE

40

SETTING

- Hospital

ETHNICITY/CULTURE

- American/Asian

PREEXISTING CONDITIONS

- Hypocalcemia

COEXISTING CONDITIONS

- Thyroidectomy X two years

LIFESTYLE

- Intake clerk

COMMUNICATION

- English as a second language

DISABILITY

SOCIOECONOMIC STATUS

- Middle

SPIRITUAL/RELIGIOUS

- Moravian

PHARMACOLOGIC

- Aluminum hydroxide (Amphogel)
- Calcitriol (Rocaltrol)

PSYCHOSOCIAL

- Anxiety

LEGAL

ETHICAL

ALTERNATIVE THERAPY

- Aerobic exercise daily
- Tai Chi

PRIORITIZATION

- Elevate serum calcium levels
- Prevent and treat convulsions
- Maintain airway patency

DELEGATION

- RN
- Client education

THE ENDOCRINE SYSTEM

Level of difficulty: Easy

Overview: This case involves a thorough assessment of the client's condition including priority care for a client experiencing signs and symptoms of hypocalcemia. The nurse must also be skilled with critical thinking to prioritize care for this client in a busy triage area. The case involves questioning the client about all drugs, including herbals, that she is currently taking.

Client Profile

Ms. J is a 40-year-old clerical "input" employee for a visiting nurse service in a busy urban area. She is brought from her place of employment to the emergency department (ED) of a busy urban hospital. On arrival she complains of numbness, tingling, and cramps in the extremities, and stiffness in the hands and feet.

Case Study

Her vital signs are:

Blood pressure: 130/80
Pulse: 78
Respirations: 18
Temperature: 98.2° F

While she is being transferred from the stretcher by an emergency medical technician (EMT), Ms. J complains of tightness in her throat, and wheezing is less audible. She is rushed into the triage area of the ED where the nurse practitioner (NP) identifies positive Trousseau's and Chvostek's signs. Stat serum calcium and phosphate levels are drawn and evaluated. The results reveal serum calcium 5 mg/dL and serum phosphate 6.5 mg/dL. On further assessment, Ms. J is less responsive and wheezing is inaudible. An emergency respiratory code is called, and the client is intubated and an intravenous line initiated with 0.9% NaCL infusion. The ED health care provider is notified, and after reviewing the NP notes and the serum calcium and phosphate levels, Ms. J is transferred to the medical intensive care unit (MICU). During transfer to MICU, Ms. J has an episode of partial seizure that lasts for two minutes. The health care provider is notified and arrives at the MICU to await the client, but the seizure subsides before the client arrives to the unit. Ms. J is given a continuous drip of 10% calcium gluconate in 1000 mLs 5% dextrose in water, infused over eight hours via an I-Med pump. A stat dose of phenytoin (Dilantin) 500 mg IV in 0.9% NaCL is also administered. An arterial blood gas (ABG) is done and reveals metabolic acidosis (pH 7.28, pO2 90, pCO_2 43, HCO_3 20) and IV sodium bicarbonate 3 mEq/kg over four hours is infused. Ms. J is responding appropriately, her breath sounds are normal, Chvostek's and Trousseau's signs are now negative, total serum calcium is 8 mg/dL, phosphorous is 4 mg/dL. ABGs are repeated and reveal: pH 7.4, pCO2 44 mm Hg, pO_2 94 mm Hg, O_2 saturation 95%, HCO_3 26 mEq/L. The client is extubated and a nasal cannula with two liters of oxygen is initiated.

Questions

1. Discuss the etiology and pathophysiology of hypoparathyroidism.

2. Discuss clinical manifestations of hypoparathyroidism.

3. Discuss the assessment and diagnostic findings of hypoparathyroidism.

4. Discuss medical and nursing management of hypoparathyroidism.

5. Discuss chronic hypoparathyroidism.

6. Discuss a critical nursing diagnosis, outcome, and interventions for hypoparathyroidism.

7. What are the purposes for the prescribed orders?

8. What are common adverse reactions, drug-to-drug, drug-to-food/herbal interactions for the prescribed medications?

9. Discuss other medications that may be used to manage hypoparathyroidism.

10. Discuss client education for hypoparathyroidism.

Questions and Suggested Answers

1. Discuss the etiology and pathophysiology of hypoparathyroidism. The most common cause of hypoparathyroidism is inadequate secretion of parathyroid hormone after interruption of the blood supply. Other causes include accidental removal of the parathyroid glands during thyroidectomy or radical neck dissection, infarction of the parathyroid glands, strangulation of one or more of the glands by postoperative scar, damage to the parathyroid tissue secondary to the removal of hyperplastic parathyroid tissue, Addison's disease, and an autoimmune response. The symptoms of hypoparathyroidism are caused by a deficiency of parathorome that results in elevated blood phosphate (hyperphosphatemia) and decreased blood calcium (hypocalcemia) levels. In the absence of parathormone, there is decreased intestinal absorption of dietary calcium and decreased resorption of calcium from bone and through the renal tubules. Decreased renal excretion of phosphate causes hypophosphaturia and low serum calcium levels, resulting in hypocalciuria.

2. Discuss clinical manifestations of hypoparathyroidism. Hypocalcemia, which causes irritability of the neuromuscular system and contributes to the chief symptom of hypoparathyroidism. Tetany (a general muscular hypertonia) with tremor and spasmodic or uncoordinated contractions occurring with or without efforts to make voluntary movements. If tetany is latent, there is numbness, tingling, and cramps in the extremities. The client usually complains of stiffness in the hands and feet. In overt tetany, the signs include bronchospasm, laryngeal spasm, carpopedal spasm (flexion of the

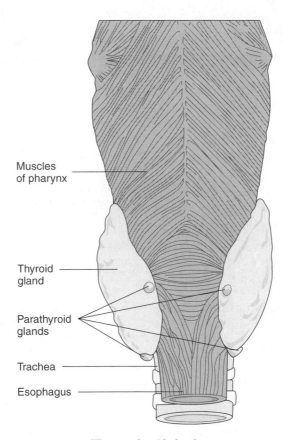

Muscles
of pharynx

Thyroid
gland

Parathyroid
glands

Trachea

Esophagus

The parathyroid glands.

elbow and wrists and extension of the carpophalangeal joints), dysphagia, photophobia, cardiac dysrhythmias, and seizures. There may be delirium, depression, electrocardiogram (EKG) changes, and hypotension.

3. Discuss the assessment and diagnostic findings of hypoparathyroidism. Latent tetany is suggested by a positive *Trousseau's sign* or a positive *Chvostek's sign.* Trousseau's sign is positive when carpopedal spasm is induced by occluding the blood flow to the arm for three minutes with the use of a blood pressure cuff. Chvostek's sign is positive when a sharp tapping over the facial nerve just in front of the parotid gland and anterior to the ear causes spasm or twitching of the mouth, nose, and eye. The diagnosis is often difficult because symptoms are usually vague (i.e., aches, pains), therefore laboratory studies are especially helpful. Tetany develops at serum calcium levels of 5–6 mg/dL. Serum phosphate levels are increased, and X-rays of bone show increased density. Calcification is detected on X-rays of subcutaneous or paraspinal basal ganglia of the brain.

4. **Discuss medical and nursing management of hypoparathyroidism.** *Medical management:* The goal of therapy is to raise the serum calcium level to 10 mg/dL and to eliminate the symptoms of hypoparathyroidism and hypocalcemia. If hypoparathyroidism is chronic (as determined by series of serum calcium levels and positive symptoms), a diet high in calcium and low in phosphorous is prescribed. Oral tablets of calcium salts, such as calcium gluconate, may supplement the diet. Aluminum hydroxide gel or aluminum carbonate (Gelusil, Amphogel) is prescribed to bind phosphate and promote its excretion through the gastrointestinal (GI) tract. The health care provider may also prescribe vitamin D preparation such as ergocalciferol or cholecalciferol to enhance calcium absorption from the GI tract. *Nursing management:* Nurses focus on monitoring the client, documenting deviated findings, and implementing orders as prescribed. Nurses work in collaboration with the certified dietitian to assure that the prescribed diet is received by the client. A diet that is low in phosphorous and high in calcium should not include increased egg yolk and spinach, because both sources are high in phosphorous and spinach contains oxalate, which would form insoluble calcium substances and raise the calcium level. A diet low in phosphorous and high in calcium would include beef, pork, dried beans, sherbet, vanilla ice cream, white or whole wheat bread, half-and-half, cottage cheese, macaroni, spaghetti, noodles, asparagus, bean sprouts, collard greens, etc. Nursing responsibilities would also include administering oral calcium salts, which should be given after meals to enhance the binding of phosphate and allow its excretion via the GI tract.

5. **Discuss chronic hypoparathyroidism.** Chronic hypoparathyroidism is usually idiopathic, resulting in lethargy; thin, patchy hair; brittle nail; dry, scaly skin; and personality changes. Ectopic or unexpected calcification may appear in the eyes and basal ganglia (the gray matter, largely composed of cell bodies, within each cerebral hemisphere), resulting in cataracts and permanent brain damage, accompanied by psychosis or convulsions. Cataracts develop from prolonged hypocalcemia, because with the decreased serum calcium, there is increased uptake of serum sodium and water by the lens of the eye, resulting in clouding or blurring of the lens. Permanent brain damage may develop from chronic hypocalcemia due to the deficit of calcium, since the body (including the brain) requires calcium ions for the transmission of nerve impulses and even a relatively small decrease in calcium can cause severe muscle contraction to organs of the body, resulting in damage. The desired outcome of intervention for chronic hypoparathyroidism is to restore the serum calcium level to normal concentrations.

6. Discuss a critical nursing diagnosis, outcome, and interventions for hypoparathyroidism.

Nursing diagnosis: risk for injury, muscle tetany R/T decreased serum calcium levels

Expected outcome: The client will be free from injury as evidenced by a return of calcium levels to normal range, a normal respiratory rate, and blood gases within normal range.

Nursing intervention: The nurse will be prepared for laryngeal spasm and respiratory obstruction by having in close proximity to the client an endotracheal tube, a laryngoscope, and a tracheostomy set. The nurse will also maintain an intravenous line readily available for rapid venous access if needed.

The following are prescribed:

- Aluminum hydroxide (Amphogel) 600 mg PO three times per day with meals
- Calcitriol (Rocaltrol) 0.25 mcg PO daily for four weeks and ergocalciferol (vitamin D_2) 25 mcg PO daily for six weeks
- Serum calcium and phosphorous levels two times per day

7. What are the purposes for the prescribed orders? *Aluminum hydroxide* and *calcitriol* are prescribed to increase the calcium levels and prevent complications. *Aluminum hydroxide* is a nonsystemic antacid that lowers serum phosphate by binding dietary phosphatase to form insoluble aluminum phosphate, which is then excreted via the feces. Because there is an inverse relationship with calcium and phosphorous, when phosphorous is decreased, calcium will be increased. *Calcitriol* is a synthetic form of an active metabolite that functions to increase sodium level by promoting intestinal absorption and renal retention of calcium and, in doing so, decreases elevated blood levels of phosphate. Monitoring serum calcium and phosphorous levels aids in the evaluation of the benefits of current medications and may rule out electrolyte imbalances. Persistent hypocalcemia adversely affects the heart, causing arrythmias that can result in cardiac failure. Persistent hyperphosphatemia can further depress the calcium level, resulting in complications.

8. What are the most common adverse reactions, drug-to-drug, drug-to-food/herbal interactions for the prescribed medications? A common adverse reaction of *aluminum hydroxide* is constipation. Drug-to-drug interactions may occur with the simultaneous use of chloroquine, cimetidine, ciprofloxacin, digoxin, isoniazid by decreasing their absorption. With the concurrent use of iron salts, nonsteroidal anti-inflammatory agents (NSAIDs), phenytoin, tetracycline, thyroxine, the development of systemic alkalosis could occur. With *aluminum hydroxide* drug-to-drug interactions may occur with the simultaneous use of allopurinol, corticosteroids, diflunisal, histamine-2 antagonists, penicillamine, thyroid hormones, ticlopidine, anticholinergics, phenothiazines, isoniazid, quinidine, phenytoin, digoxin iron salts, warfarin, ketoconazole, or ciprofloxacin, because aluminum hydroxide decreases the effectiveness of these agents, requiring an increase in their dosages unless administration is separated by at least two hours. If quinidine, mexiletine, tetracyclines, and sodium polystyrene sulfonate are used simultaneously with aluminum hydroxide there is an increased risk of systemic alkalosis. There are no clinically significant drug-to-food/herbal interactions established. The most common adverse effects of *calcitriol* include drowsiness, headache, nausea and palpitations. Drug-to-drug interactions may occur with the simultaneous use of *calcitriol* and cholestyramine, mineral oil, and fat-soluble vitamins that can decrease the absorption of calcitriol. Hypercalcemia can occur with the concurrent use of thiazide diuretics and calcium supplements. Cardiac dysrythmias may result from the simultaneous use of cardiac glycosides or verapamil. Phenytoin increases the metabolism of vitamin D. Drug-to-food interactions may result if the client eats large amounts of high-calcium foods (dark-green leafy vegetables, sardines, and blackstrap molasses), causing hypercalcemia. No clinically significant drug-to-herbal interactions have been established. Drug-to-drug interactions may occur with the simultaneous use of *ergocalciferol* and cholestyramine, colestipol, and mineral oil, which may decrease its absorption. There are no clinically significant drug-to-food/herbal interactions established.

9. **Discuss other medications that may be used to manage hypoparathyroidism.** *Calcium gluconate 10%*, if prescribed, is administered in intravenous solution (0.9% NaCL) to elevate serum calcium levels quickly if the condition is acute, but its mechanism of action is not clear. When the situation is stabilized and the danger of tetany has passed, oral calcium is prescribed and implemented to maintain normal serum calcium levels. The client is also given vitamin D (ergocalciferol) to aid in the increase and stabilization of serum calcium levels.

10. Discuss client education for hypoparathyroidism. The client should be instructed that foods high in calcium and low in phosphorous will increase calcium level while decreasing the phosphorous level. Foods high in calcium are dark-green leafy vegetables, sardines, and blackstrap molasses. Calcium and vitamin D are best absorbed in an acidic environment. Therefore, the client may add lemon juice to vegetables. Dark-green leafy vegetables help to facilitate calcium absorption. Foods that are high in magnesium should be included in the diet because magnesium levels are usually low in hypoparathyroidism, and magnesium is needed to help increase the absorption of calcium. Foods high in magnesium include peanut butter, milk, chicken (dark, roasted without the skin), beef liver, oatmeal, whole wheat bread, boiled spinach, baked sweet potato, raisins, orange juice, and cheddar cheese. Aluminum hydroxide should be taken with meals.

References

Broyles, B. E. (2005). *Medical-Surgical Nursing Clinical Companion*. Durham, NC: Carolina Academic Press.

Corbet, J. V. (2004). *Laboratory Tests and Diagnostic Procedures with Nursing Diagnoses* (6th ed.). Upper Saddle River, NJ: Prentice Hall.

Gahart, B. L. and Nazareno, A. R. (2005). *2005 Intravenous Medications*. St. Louis: Mosby.

Heitz, U. and Horne, M. M. (2005). *Mosby's Pocket Guide Series: Fluid, Electrolyte and Acid-Base Balance* (5th ed.). St. Louis: Mosby.

Huether, S. E. and McCance, K. L. (2004). *Understanding Pathophysiology* (3rd ed.). St. Louis: Mosby.

Ignatavicius, D. D. and Workman, M. L. (2006). *Medical-Surgical Nursing across the Health Care Continuum* (5th ed.). Philadelphia: W. B. Saunders.

Spratto, G. R. and Woods, A. L. (2005). *2005 Edition: PDR Nurse's Drug Handbook*. Clifton Park, NY: Thomson Delmar Learning.

Hyperparathyroidism

E A S Y

GENDER

F

AGE

68

SETTING

- Hospital

ETHNICITY/CULTURE

- Hispanic/American

PREEXISTING CONDITIONS

- Osteoporosis

COEXISTING CONDITIONS

- Recent fracture of lower extremity

LIFESTYLE

- Retired principal, elementary school

COMMUNICATION

- English and Spanish

DISABILITY

- Cardiac compromise resulted in early retirement

SOCIOECONOMIC STATUS

- Middle

SPIRITUAL/RELIGIOUS

- Evangelical

PHARMACOLOGIC

- Furosemide (Lasix)
- Plicamycin (Mithracin)

PSYCHOSOCIAL

- Anxiety

LEGAL

ETHICAL

- Clients have the right to use homeopathic remedies with prescribed medical regimen.

ALTERNATIVE THERAPY

- Homeopathic medicine: feverfew, vitamin C, folic acid, and thiamine
- Meditation

PRIORITIZATION

- Reduce serum calcium levels
- Increase phosphorous

DELEGATION

- RN
- Client education

THE ENDOCRINE SYSTEM

Level of difficulty: Easy

Overview: This case involves a thorough assessment of the client's condition, including pre-scribed drugs and herbals the client is presently taking. It involves prioritization in a triage sit-uation with appropriate delegation of personnel to stabilize and maintain the client's fluid and electrolyte status. It also involves questioning the client about symptoms, bone fractures, recent weight loss, arthritis, and history of radiation treatment.

Client Profile

Mrs. R had just returned from vacation with her husband and grandchildren when she accidentally fell climbing the stairs to their bedroom. She is taken to the hospital emergency department (ED) by her husband. On arrival the client complains of pain of the right hip and shoulders. While being triaged, Mrs. R reports previous falls and fractures, frequent constipation, and epigastric discomfort.

Case Study

Mrs. R is seen by the ED health care provider, and after history, physical, and complete assessment, the health care provider orders computed tomography (CT) scan of the head and long bones, X-rays of the lower extremities and shoulders, and X-rays of the kidneys. Mrs. R is transferred from the radiology department to the orthopedic unit and is placed on bed rest, with continued nursing assessment done by a registered nurse (RN). Mrs. R reports fatigue and weight loss prior to leaving for vacation and emphasized that even though her appetite was better during the vacation, she was still fatigued and lost three pounds within a two-week period while on vacation. Magnetic resonance imaging (MRI) reveals beginning hyperplasia of the parathyroid gland. Bone scan shows bone demineralization of the lower extremities and contusion of the left ankle. The head and shoulders are normal as revealed by the CT scan. X-ray of the kidneys reveals kidney stones but no abnormalities in the bones or soft tissues. Ultrasonography supports renal calculi in the right kidney. Serum lab results drawn in the ED reveal total serum calcium 12.0 mg/dl, phosphorous 2.0 mg/dL and serum PTH levels 68 pg/mL and total urine and serum cyclic AMP excretion levels increased. After the health care provider reviews the results of diagnostic and lab tests, a diagnosis of primary hyperparathyroidism is confirmed. Mrs. R is placed on telemetry and seizure precaution. Serum calcium and phosphorous will be monitored daily, as ordered.

Questions

1. Discuss the etiology, risk factors, incidence, and pathophysiology of hyperparathyroidism.

2. Discuss major clinical manifestations for hyperparathyroidism.

3. Discuss diagnostic studies for hyperparathyroidism.

4. Discuss nursing diagnoses for hyperparathyroidism.

5. Discuss complications of hyperparathyroidism.

6. Discuss the relationship of excess parathyroid hormone (PTH) and bone damage.

Questions (continued)

7. What are the purposes for the pre-scribed orders?

8. What are the most common adverse reactions, drug-to-drug, drug-to-food/herbal interactions of the prescribed medications?

9. Discuss hydration and diet therapy for hyperparathyroidism.

10. Discuss client education for hyperparathyroidism.

Questions and Suggested Answers

1. **Discuss the etiology, risk factors, incidence, and pathophysiology of hyperparathyroidism.** Hyperparathyroidism is classified as primary, secondary, or tertiary. *Primary* hyperparathyroidism is due to an increased secretion of parathyroid hormone (PTH) leading to disorders of calcium, phosphate, and bone metabolism. It is more common in women and usually occurs between 30 and 70 years of age. The peak incidence is in the fifth and sixth decades of life. People who have previously undergone head and neck radiation may have an increased predisposition to the development of parathyroid ade-noma. *Secondary* hyperparathyroidism is believed to be a compensatory response to states that induce or cause hypocalcemia, the main stimulus for PTH secretion. Disease conditions associated with secondary hyperparathy-roidism include vitamin D deficiency, malabsorption, chronic renal failure, and hyperphosphatemia. *Tertiary* hyperparathyroidism occurs when there is hyperplasia of the parathyroid glands and a loss of negative feedback from cir-culating calcium levels. The result is autonomous secretion of PTH, even with normal calcium levels. The pathophysiology is seen when circulating levels of PTH cause hypercalcemia and hypophosphatemia, creating a multisystem effect. In the bones, subperiosteal bone resorption, decreased bone density, cyst formation, and general weakness due to the effect of PTH on osteoclastic (bone resorption) and osteoblastic (bone formation) activity. In the kidneys, the excess calcium cannot be reabsorbed, leading to increased levels of calcium in the urine (hypercalciuria). The urinary calcium and the large amounts of urinary phosphate can lead to urinary calculi formation. In addi-tion, PTH stimulates the simulator of calcium transport in the intestine, thereby indirectly increasing gastrointestinal (GI) absorption of calcium, contributing further to the high serum calcium levels.

2. **Discuss major clinical manifestations of hyperparathyroidism.** The major manifestations include weakness, loss of appetite, constipation, increased need for sleep, emotional disorders, and shortened attention span. Major signs include loss of calcium from the bones (osteoporosis), fractures, and kidney stones (nephrolithiasis).

3. **Discuss diagnostic studies for hyperparathyroidism.** PTH level as measured by radioimmunoassay and is elevated, and serum calcium levels that usually exceed 10 mg/dL, with the serum phosphorous level usually low, below 3 mg/dL. Other labs that are usually elevated are urine calcium, serum chloride, uric acid, creatinine, and alkaline phosphatase (in the presence of bone disease).

4. **Discuss nursing diagnoses for hyperparathyroidism.**
- High risk for injury R/T demineralization of bones – Health care providers will provide a safe environment for the client at all times. Bed should be kept in low position and side rails in upright position and locked. Client should be turned and positioned gently to prevent pathologic fractures.
- Impaired urinary elimination R/T renal involvement secondary to hypercalcemia – Health care providers should monitor urinary output, maintain accurate intake and output, document and report deviation from normal. Appropriate skin care to prevent breakdown from dehydration.
- Constipation related to GI hypomotility R/T adverse effects of hypercalcemia on the GI tract – Nursing care will focus on assessment of bowel pattern and characteristics of stools to plan appropriate interventions. Administer medications as prescribed to decrease calcium level and maintain calcium balance. Provision of two to three liters of fluids per day to maintain soft stool. Offer foods high in bulk and roughage to increase fecal mass. Encourage activity to stimulate peristalsis.
- Decreased thought processes R/T diminished cerebral blood flow secondary to effects of hypercalcemia – The nurse will assess thinking processes such as memory, attention span, and orientation to enable appropriate planning. Health care providers will repeat information to client and allow quality time to process and comprehend information. Provide clock and calendar to maintain reality orientation to time and day.
- Knowledge deficit R/T condition, treatment, and health maintenance – The nurse will explain to the client the signs and symptoms of the disease process and emphasize the importance of reporting unusual signs and symptoms promptly to the health care provider. Handouts that are written in understandable language should accompany verbal instructions.

5. **Discuss complications of hyperparathyroidism.** Complications of hyperparathyroidism include *renal failure* and *pancreatitis. Renal failure* results when the kidneys are unable to remove the body's metabolic wastes or perform their regulatory functions. *Renal failure* may develop from hyperparathyroidism because of the calcium abnormalities (renal calculi), initially resulting in urolithiasis. Most (75–80%) kidney stones are calcium stones, composed of calcium oxalate and/or calcium phosphate as seen with hyperparathyroidism. Stones can obstruct the urinary tract at any point from the calyces of the kidney to the distal urethra, impeding the outflow of the urine. Urinary tract obstruction can ultimately lead to stasis then infection as the stones gradually damage the urethra, and eventually renal failure develops. The amount of urine output helps determine possible urinary tract obstruction and adequacy of hydration. Dysuria, frequency, urgency, and cloudy urine are symptoms of urinary tract infection often associated with urolithiasis. As the pathology progresses, urinary output will further decrease; blood urea nitrogen (BUN) and creatinine levels will increase. If pharmacologic interventions and invasive procedures do not correct the problems, peritoneal dialysis or hemodialysis will be initiated to maintain quality of life by removing waste products from the body that the kidneys are not able to perform. *Pancreatitis* occurs secondary to hypercalcemia and is one of the manifestations of the disease processes. Acute pancreatitis could develop due to intravascular volume depletion (polyuria). When there is severe volume depletion, there is blockage of the main secretory duct of the pancreas, as well as the common bile duct. Eventually, the pancreatic enzymes are dammed up in the ducts and acini of the pancreas, resulting in inflammation of the pancreas.

6. **Discuss the relationship of excess parathyroid hormone (PTH) and bone damage.** The oversecretion of PTH causes excessive osteoclast growth and activity within the bones. Osteoclasts promote resorption of bone, and when bone resorption is increased, calcium is released from the bones into the blood, causing hypercalcemia. When hypercalcemia develops, the bones become demineralized because of the calcium loss, and if not corrected, it results in fragility of the bones and the development of pathologic bone changes and bone damage. When there is excessive PTH, it causes hyperphosphaturia, and as serum calcium continues to rise in hyperparathyroidism, excessive amounts of both phosphorous and calcium are excreted and lost from the body. Large amounts of calcium and phosphorous are excreted by the renal systems. If tumor is the cause of the excess production of PTH and surgery is not done, renal disease develops and may be irreversible.

The following are prescribed:

- IV 0.9% normal saline infusion at 125 mLs/hr
- Furosemide (Lasix) 40 mg IV stat then 80 mg q8h × 24 hours
- Plicamycin (Mithracin) 10 mg/kg of body weight IV × two via slow infusion
- Serum calcium, phosphate, and sodium levels two times per day

7. **What are the purposes for the prescribed orders?** *Intravenous fluid* of normal saline should be administered concomitantly with intravenous furosemide to maintain hydration and aid with the excretion of serum calcium. *Furosemide* is a loop diuretic that causes diuresis to aid in the over-excretion of calcium in the urine. It works by inhibiting resorption of sodium and chloride in Henle's loop and, in doing so, enhances diuresis and elimination of the excess calcium. *Plicamycin* is an antihypercalcemic and antineoplastic that lowers serum calcium by inhibiting bone resorption. Serum calcium, phosphate, and sodium levels need to be monitored to determine the effectiveness of treatment and to determine a potential adverse effect of normal saline intravenous administration.

8. **What are the most common adverse reactions, drug-to-drug, drug-to-food/herbal interactions of the prescribed medications?** The primary adverse effect associated with *0.9% normal saline* intravenous infusion is hypernatremia. Although this solution is isotonic in nature, it can aggravate existing acidosis, anorexia, cellular dehydration, edema, hydrogen loss, hypertension, hypokalemia, fluid overload, and weakness. The most common adverse reactions of *furosemide* are hypotension, hypokalemia, hyperuricemia, hyponatremia, and hyperchloremia. The most common adverse reactions of *plicamycin* are stomatitis, anorexia, nausea, vomiting, hypocalcemia, thrombocytopenia, and diarrhea. There are few drug-to-drug interactions with *0.9% sodium chloride infusion*. Mannitol is not compatible with this solution and will cause phlebitis if infused with normal saline. No clinically significant drug-to-food/herbal interactions have been established, although foods high in sodium will increase the risk of hypernatremia and fluid overload. Drug-to-drug interactions may occur with the simultaneous use of *furosemide* and other diuretics that may enhance diuretic effects and increase the risk of toxicity. It potentiates the effects of antihypertensive agents and anticoagulants. It may increase the serum levels of beta blockers and lithium. The simultaneous use with amphotericin B, stimulant laxatives, and corticosteroids potentiate hypokalemia, and its simultaneous use with insulin or sulfonylurease may mask the effects of hyperglycemia, and with aminoglycosides or ethacrynic acid furosemide, markedly increases the risk of ototoxicity. It may enhance or inhibit the actions of nondepolarizing muscle relaxants or theophyllines. Furosemide is inhibited by angiotensin-converting enzyme (ACE) inhibitors, nonsteroidal anti-inflammatory agents (NSAIDs), phenytoin, and salicylates. When administered intravenously, each 40 mg or less should be administered over one to two minutes. There are no clinically significant drug-to-food/herbal interactions established.

With *plicamycin* drug-to-drug interactions may occur with the simultaneous use of vitamin D, which may enhance hypercalcemia and increase the risk of bleeding with the simultaneous use of aspirin, NSAIDs, dipyridamole, warfarin, thrombolytic agents, heparin, cephalosporins, ticlopidine, clopidogrel, tirofiban, eptifibatide, valproic acid, dextran, or sulfinpyrazone. Additive myelosuppression with other antineoplastics may occur with the simultaneous use of plicamycin. Increased risk of nephrotoxicity occurs with the concurrent use of plicamycin and acyclovir, aminoglycosides, and amphotericin B. It may be antagonized by calcium or vitamin D supplements. Drug-to-food interactions are not clinically established. Drug-to-herbal interactions are seen with the simultaneous use of anise, arnica, chamomile, clove, dong quai, tenugreek, feverfew, garlic, ginger, gingko, Panax ginseng, and licorice.

9. **Discuss hydration and diet therapy for hyperparathyroidism.** The nurse will encourage intake of foods low in calcium to help correct the hypercalcemia; explain to the client that omission of milk and milk products from meals may help decrease some of the GI symptoms (e.g., anorexia and nausea); assess location, duration, and intensity of pain; administer pain medication on time as scheduled; monitor hydration therapy hourly; encourage increase in fluid intake; monitor intake and output, and strain all urine; document constituents of urine; monitor serum calcium, phosphate, and sodium levels; explain rationale for treatment plan to client.

10. **Discuss client education for hyperparathyroidism.** Limit carbonated beverages, because they are high in phosphates and may decrease calcium absorption. Avoid coffee, black tea, colas, and chocolate, as these can lead to further calcium loss. Emphasize the benefits of small frequent feedings, because anorexia is a common occurrence. Prune juice, stool softeners, physical activity, and increased fluid intake will help to offset constipation. Compliance with prescribed orders is important so that calcium and phosphorous levels can be measured to ascertain that they are within normal limits.

References

Corbet, J. V. (2004). *Laboratory Tests and Diagnostic Procedures with Nursing Diagnoses* (6th ed.). Upper Saddle River, NJ: Prentice Hall.

Decker, G. M. (April/March 2003). "Commonly Used Vitamin Supplements: Implications for Clinical Practice." *Clinical Journal of Oncology Nursing* 7(2): 1–28.

Drezner, M. K., Neelon, F. A., Curtis, H. B., and Lebovitz, H. E. (2004). "Renal Cyclic Adenosine Monophosphate: An Accurate Index of Parathyroid Function." Available at www.ncbi.nlm.nih.gov.

Huether, S. E. and McCance, K. L. (2004). *Understanding Pathophysiology* (3rd ed.). St. Louis: Mosby.

Ignatavicius, D. D. and Workman, M. L. (2006). *Medical-Surgical Nursing across the Health Care Continuum* (5th ed.). Philadelphia: W. B. Saunders.

Spratto, G. R. and Woods, A. L. (2005). *2005 Edition: PDR Nurse's Drug Handbook.* Clifton Park, NY: Thomson Delmar Learning.

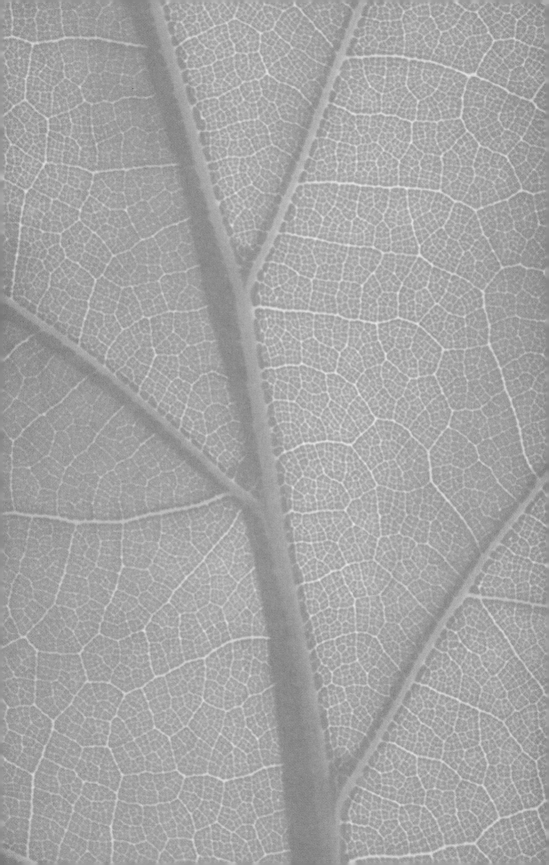

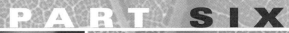

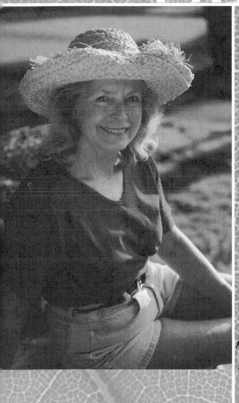

PART SIX

*The Musculoskeletal
and Reproductive
Systems*

CASE STUDY 1

Benign Prostatic Hypertrophy

GENDER

M

AGE

58

SETTING

- Urology clinic

ETHNICITY/CULTURE

- Black American

PREEXISTING CONDITIONS

- Prostatis
- Urinary tract infection

COEXISTING CONDITIONS

- Mild urinary frequency
- Dysuria

LIFESTYLE

- Licensed plumber

COMMUNICATION

DISABILITY

SOCIOECONOMIC STATUS

- Middle

SPIRITUAL/RELIGIOUS

- Methodist

PHARMACOLOGIC

- Finasteride (Proscar)
- Terazosin (Hytrin)
- Saw palmetto

PSYCHOSOCIAL

- Anxiety

LEGAL

ETHICAL

- The right to use herbal medicine
- The surgeon needs to provide a clear and simple explanation of what the procedure will entail, the benefits, alternatives, risks, and complications.

ALTERNATIVE THERAPY

- Saw palmetto

PRIORITIZATION

- Relieve bladder distention
- Improve urinary flow

DELEGATION

- RN
- Client education

THE MUSCULOSKELETAL AND REPRODUCTIVE SYSTEMS

Level of difficulty: Easy

Overview: This case involves a thorough assessment of the client's condition, with focus on urinary pattern and any experience with hematuria. It also involves questioning the client about medications presently being used, since drugs such as anticholinergics, antihistamines, and decongestions can cause urinary retention. The nurse should be skilled at assessing clients with risk for urinary alteration, to prevent urinary complications.

Client Profile

Mr. C is a 48-year-old male who has had no medical or surgical history until the last two months when he noticed a change in his urinary flow accompanied with burning and incomplete bladder emptying. After sharing his concerns with a male registered nurse (RN) in the neighborhood, Mr. C was encouraged to seek medical advice.

Case Study

Mr. C is seen by a health care provider in the urology clinic of the community hospital. On initial interview, Mr. C reports urinary frequency and urgency over the past two weeks and emphasized how annoying the symptoms were. On routine examination, the health care provider finds a prostate gland that is large, rubbery, and non-tender. On direct rectal examination (DRE) the prostate is symmetrically enlarged, firm, and smooth. His respiratory status is normal as revealed by pulmonary function studies and physical assessment. His cardiac status is normal as evidenced by normal sinus rhythm seen on electrocardiogram (EKG) and a normal echocardiogram revealing normal structures of the heart. His vital signs are:

Blood pressure: 140/78
Pulse: 80
Respirations: 14
Temperature: 98.4° F

The health care provider reviews the plan of care with Mr. C, and prescriptions for serum and urinalysis laboratory tests are given. He will take a sterile urine specimen for urinalysis to a specified lab in his community to be analyzed.

At the lab Mr. C has blood specimens drawn for white blood cell (WBC) count, blood urea nitrogen (BUN), creatinine, and serum for prostatic-specific antigen (PSA) level. He schedules a second blood specimen to be drawn by the lab. Those results will be sent to the health care provider and reviewed on Mr. C's next scheduled visit. Mr. C is also scheduled for a transurethral ultrasound (TRUS) scan at a community diagnostic center. These results will also be sent to the health care provider. Upon return to his health care provider for follow-up visits, the results of the labs and diagnostic tests are discussed with Mr. C. The test results reveal:

Urinalysis: negative
Blood urea nitrogen (BUN): 20 mg/dL

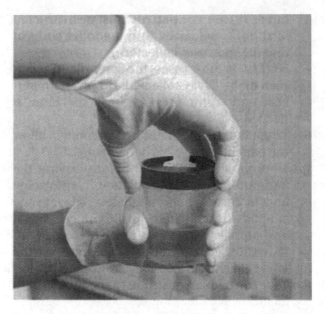

Care must be taken in the handling of bodily fluids to prevent the transfer of infectious agents through contact with secretions.

Creatinine: 1.2 mg/dL
Repeat PSA level: 5.8 ng/mL

The TRUS reveals an enlarged prostate with small fibrous nodules but no obstruction of urethra flow. A diagnosis of benign prostatic hypertrophy is confirmed, and a treatment plan is discussed with Mr. C.

Questions

1. Discuss the incidence, etiology, risk factors, and pathophysiology of benign prostatic hyperplasia (BPH).

2. Discuss the difference between prostate cancer and BPH.

3. Discuss clinical manifestations of BPH.

4. Discuss diagnostic findings in BPH.

5. What are the purposes for the prescribed medications?

6. What are the most common adverse reactions, drug-to-drug, drug-to-food/herbal interactions of the prescribed medications?

7. Discuss phytotherapeutic agents (the use of herbs for healing purposes) for BPH.

8. Discuss complications of BPH.

9. Discuss intermittent self-catheterization for men with BPH.

10. Discuss client education for BPH.

Questions and Suggested Answers

1. **Discuss the incidence, etiology, risk factors, and pathophysiology of benign prostatic hyperplasia (BPH).** BPH is the most common benign tumor of the prostate gland. The incidence of BPH consistently increases with age, and it is estimated that by 50 years of age, 50% of men have some degree of BPH. The incidence increases with each decade of life, and of men over 80 years of age, approximately 90% have BPH. The exact cause of BPH is not known, but factors such as diet, effects of chronic inflammation, socioeconomic factors, heredity, and race have all been considered. Testicular androgen seems to be the most common hormone suspected as a cause of BPH. Obesity, particularly an increased abdominal girth, is a contributing factor. Aging is a major risk factor for the development of BPH, so there are no primary preventions. However, early detection is the best secondary prevention. Benign prostatic enlargement occurs by an abnormal increase in the number of normal cells (hyperplasia) in the prostate, rather than an increase in cell size (hypertrophy). With aging, the periurethral glands undergo hyperplasia, and gradually they grow and compress surrounding normal prostatic tissue, pushing it toward the gland periphery, forming a false capsule.

2. **Discuss the difference between BHP and prostate cancer.**

Benign Prostatic Hypertrophy	Prostate Cancer
Incidence	**Incidence**
More common in white males in the United States.	More common in African Americans in the world.
Increase in age is a risk factor	Increase in age is a risk factor. Risk increases rapidly after the age of 50.
Alteration in urinary elimination is a common problem. PSA (increased) and rectal examination and prostatic massage aids in confirmation of BPH.	PSA used as a tumor marker, and needle aspiration or biopsy used to confirm suspected malignancy.
Complications	**Complications**
Hydronephrosis	Sexual dysfunction is common even before the diagnosis is determined.
Urinary obstruction	
Urinary retention	

3. **Discuss clinical manifestations of BPH.** The common physical assessment finding is a large prostate gland that is rubbery and nontender, probably due to hormones causing hyperplasia of the supporting stromal tissue and the glandular elements in the prostate. Other findings include urinary frequency and urgency, urinary incontinence, weak stream of urine when

urinating, terminal dribbling, and intermittent interruption in the urine stream, nocturia, dysuria, and urinary retention. Abdominal straining with urination, a decrease in volume and a force of the urinary stream.

4. **Discuss diagnostic findings in BPH.** DRE is performed to assess the prostate size and to differentiate BPH from prostate enlargement related to adenocarcinoma. BPH will reveal a symmetrically enlarged prostate with an obliterated central sulcus. PSA is done to rule out the presence of cancer. The normal level is <2.8 ng/mL; elevation indicates the presence of prostate cancer, although increased values have been noted in bladder as well as in prostatic carcinoma. Therefore, increased levels of PSA correlate with the amount of prostatic tissue, both malignant and benign.

The following are prescribed:

- Finasteride (Proscar) 5 mg PO daily
- Terazosin (Hytrin) 1 mg PO daily
- 'Client may continue to use saw palmetto (*Serenoa repens*).'

5. **What are the purposes for the prescribed medications?** *Finasteride* is an androgen hormone inhibitor that lowers the level of dihydrotesterone (DHT), which is a major cause of prostate growth. It acts by blocking the enzyme 5-a-Reductase, which is necessary for the conversion of testosterone to dihydroxytestosterone, the principal intraprostatic androgen. Finasteride causes regression of hyperplastic tissue through suppression of androgens. *Terazosin* is an alpha-1-adrenergic blocking agent that reduces urethral pressure and improves urine flow by selecting blocking alpha$_1$-adrenergic receptors in vascular smooth muscle, producing relaxation that leads to reduction of peripheral vascular resistance, thus enhancing blood flow throughout the structures of the kidneys.

6. **What are the most common adverse reactions, drug-to-drug, drug-to-food/herbal interactions of the prescribed medications?** Adverse effects associated with *finasteride* include impotence, decreased libido, decreased volume of ejaculation, testicular pain, and the potential for hypersensitivity reactions. When used with terazosin, there are increased serum levels of finasteride. There are no clinically significant drug-to-food interactions of finasteride. Drug-to-herbal interactions may occur with the simultaneous use of saw palmetto, which may potentiate the effects of finasteride. The most common adverse reactions of *terazosin* occur with the first dose and include dizziness, headache, weakness, nasal congestion, marked orthostatic hypotension, and nausea. Drug-to-drug interactions may occur with the simultaneous use of antihypertensives, which may increase hypotensive effects, or the use with nonsteroidal anti-inflammatory agents (NSAIDs), nitrates, and sympathomimetics or estrogens may decrease the effects of

antihypertensive agents. There are no clinically significant drug-to-food/herbal interactions established.

7. **Discuss phytotherapeutic agents (the use of herbs for healing purposes) for BPH.** The most widely used agent is *Serenoa repens* (saw palmetto), an antiadrogen herb. Its principal action in relationship to BPH appears to be inhibition of 5-alpha reductase enzyme activities, similar to the action of finasteride. 5-alpha-reductase enzyme inhibitors slow prostate growth by inhibiting the conversion of testosterone into DHT in the prostate gland. Adverse effects include headache, nausea, vomiting, anorexia, constipation, diarrhea, abdominal pain, dysuria, impotence, urinary retention, back pain, and hypersensitivity. Drug interactions will occur with the simultaneous use of anticoagulants by increasing the anticoagulant effects; with antiplatelets and nonsteroidal agents (NSAIDs), increased bleeding time may occur.

8. **Discuss complications for BPH.** *Hydronephrosis* or distention of the pelvis and calyces of the kidney by urine that cannot flow past an obstruction in a ureter is one of the complications of BPH. The client experiences pain in the flank and, in some cases, hematuria, pyuria, and hyperpyrexia. The health care provider may order an intravenous pyelogram, cystoscopy, or a retrograde pyelography to confirm the diagnosis. Surgical repair or removal of the obstruction may be necessary. Prolonged hydronephrosis causes atrophy and eventual loss of kidney function. *Impeded outflow of urine* is another complication of BPH. It results in ascending urinary tract infection. Management involves identifying then eliminating the cause. If signs of infection are present, gram stain of the urine is done to identify the infected organism classification, and urine culture and sensitivity test is done to identify the organism and the most effective antibiotic.

9. **Discuss intermittent self-catheterization for men with BPH.** The use of intermittent self-catheterization is indicated if the client is experiencing transient or persistent urinary retention. An indwelling catheter is not used for the procedure, therefore clients must have sufficient manual dexterity and cognitive ability, and should be able to follow guidelines. Catheterization should be done at least four times per day to prevent the urinary bladder from overfilling, since persistent overfilling can cause ureterovesical reflux with subsequent renal damage. Although self-catheterization is not a sterile procedure, medical asepsis must be maintained with good hand-washing and care of the catheter after each use.

10. **Discuss client education for BPH.** The client should have annual DREs and PSA tests. The client should comply with instructions for follow-up care. The client should communicate with health care provider about the intent to use herbal medicine as an alternate means.

References

Black, J. M. and Hawks, J. H. (2005). *Medical-Surgical Nursing: Clinical Management for Positive Outcomes* (7th ed.). St. Louis: Mosby.

Broyles, B. E. (2005). *Medical-Surgical Nursing Clinical Companion.* Durham, NC: Carolina Academic Press.

Corbet, J. V. (2004). *Laboratory Tests and Diagnostic Procedures with Nursing Diagnoses* (6th ed.). Upper Saddle River, NJ: Prentice Hall.

Deglin, J. H. and Vallerand, A. H. (2005). *Davis's Drug Guide for Nurses* (9th ed.). Philadelphia: F. A. Davis.

Gahart, B. L. and Nazareno, A. R. (2005). *2005 Intravenous Medications.* St. Louis: Elsevier Mosby.

Heitz, U. and Horne, M. M. (2005). *Mosby's Pocket Guide Series: Fluid, Electrolyte and Acid-Base Balance* (5th ed.). St. Louis: Mosby.

Huether, S. E. and McCance, K. L. (2004). *Understanding Pathophysiology* (3rd ed.). St. Louis: Mosby.

Ignatavicius, D. D. and Workman, M. L. (2006). *Medical-Surgical Nursing across the Health Care Continuum* (5th ed.). Philadelphia: W. B. Saunders.

"Prostate Problems: Facts, Disease Prevention, and Treatment Strategies." (July 2005). Available at www.healingwithnutrition.com/pdisease/prostate/prostate.html.

Skidmore-Roth, L. (2006). *Mosby's Handbook of Herbs & Natural Supplements* (3rd ed.). St. Louis: Mosby.

Spratto, G. R. and Woods, A. L. (2005). *2005 Edition: PDR Nurse's Drug Handbook.* Clifton Park, NY: Thomson Delmar Learning.

CASE STUDY 2

Ovarian Cancer

GENDER

F

AGE

42

SETTING

- Outpatient clinic of hospital

ETHNICITY/CULTURE

- White American

PREEXISTING CONDITIONS

COEXISTING CONDITIONS

- Cervical dysplasia

LIFESTYLE

- Housewife

COMMUNICATION

DISABILITY

SOCIOECONOMIC STATUS

- Middle

SPIRITUAL/RELIGIOUS

- Episcopalian

PHARMACOLOGIC

- Cisplatin (Platinol)
- Paclitaxel (Taxol)
- Aprepitant (Emend)

PSYCHOSOCIAL

- Anxiety
- Fear

LEGAL

ETHICAL

ALTERNATIVE THERAPY

- Meditation
- Aloe vera

PRIORITIZATION

- Assess for abdominal pain, heavy menstrual flow
- Palpation for abdominal mass
- Prepare for diagnostic tests

DELEGATION

- RN
- Client education

MODERATE

THE MUSCULOSKELETAL AND REPRODUCTIVE SYSTEMS

Level of difficulty: Moderate

Overview: This case involves a thorough history and physical of the client's condition including past medical, surgical, and family history. The use of active listening and critical thinking skills is needed to effectively gather data and implement therapeutic plan of care.

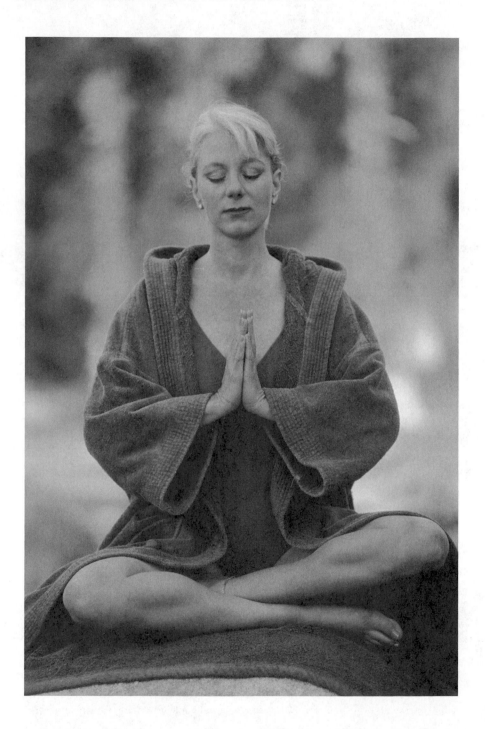

Client Profile

Mrs. E is a 42-year-old married woman and a mother of one child who is two-and-a-half years old. Mrs. E is 5'10" and weighs 182 pounds. She is accompanied by her husband of four years (who is an engineer employed by an electrical company) to her GYN health care provider due to complaints of irregular menses and increasing menorrhagia and breast tenderness.

Case Study

Mrs. E also reports flatulence, fatigue, bloating, fullness after a light meal, and constipation with increase in her abdominal girth. During the interview she is anxious and relates the anxiety to a family history of cancer. (Her mother died of breast cancer at age 78, and her older sister died of cervical cancer at age 52.) She reports that she practices meditation to relieve anxiety. After a routine examination by the GYN health care provider, Mrs. E is referred to the hospital for admission and further evaluation. Mrs. E reports yearly Pap smears and mammography, and monthly breast self-examination (BSE). She brings to the hospital a copy of a most recent report of abnormal Pap smears × 2. Her vital signs on admission are:

Blood pressure: 130/78
Pulse: 78 and regular
Respirations: 20
Temperature: 98.6° F

Mrs. E is triaged in the emergency department (ED) and transferred to the medical unit, to the GYN service where she is interviewed by a nurse practitioner (NP) and a history and physical is done. A computed tomography (CT) scan of the abdomen and ovary is ordered and detects a tumor on the right ovary that is 8 cm. A barium enema is also ordered and is negative for tumors of adjacent structures. A chest X-ray is negative for pleural effusion. Mrs. E is informed of the findings of the CT and barium enema by the NP and is later seen by a GYN health care provider, who reinforces the findings of the diagnostic tests. Serum labs are ordered: Na, K+, Hct, Hgb, WBC, platelet count (PLT), urinalysis, type and cross match for two units of packed red blood cells (PRBCs). The results of the labs are:

Sodium (Na): 138
Potassium (K+): 4
Hematocrit (Hct): 28%
Hemoglobin (Hgb): 14 g/dL
White blood cell (WBC) count: 10,000
Platelet count (PLT): 150,000
Urinalysis: negative

After the labs are reviewed, the GYN health care provider, NP, and oncologist in collaboration with Mrs. E decide to treat the tumor with cancer chemotherapy agents and blood transfusion because of her low hematocrit level.

Questions

1. Discuss the etiology and pathophysiology of ovarian cancer.

2. Discuss the incidence of ovarian cancer.

3. Discuss clinical manifestations of ovarian cancer.

4. Discuss diagnostic studies to confirm ovarian cancer.

5. What are the purposes for the prescribed orders?

6. What are the most common adverse reactions, drug-to-drug, drug-to-

food/herbal interactions of the prescribed medications?

7. Describe the various staging done with ovarian cancer.

8. Discuss surgical management of ovarian malignancy.

9. Discuss client education for ovarian cancer.

10. Explain clinical implications for ovarian cancer.

Questions and Suggested Answers

1. **Discuss the etiology and pathophysiology of ovarian cancer.** Ovarian cancer is a malignant neoplasm of the ovaries. It is the fifth leading cause of cancer deaths in the United States, and because most women with ovarian cancer have advanced disease at time of diagnosis, it causes more deaths than any other cancer of the female reproductive system. The cause of ovarian cancer varies, but studies have shown that women who have mutations of the BRCA genes have increased susceptibility for ovarian cancer. The BRCA genes are tumor suppressor genes that inhibit tumor growth when functioning normally. When these genes mutate, they lose their tumor-suppressor ability, resulting in increased risk for the development of ovarian cancer.

2. **Discuss the incidence of ovarian cancer.** About 10% of cases of ovarian cancer are genetically related. Women with BRCA-1 mutations have a 25–40% lifetime risk for developing ovarian cancer. Family history of both breast and ovarian cancer increases the risk of having a BRCA mutation. BRCA mutations occur in 10–20% of clients with ovarian cancer who have no family history of breast or ovarian cancer.

3. **Discuss clinical manifestations of ovarian cancer.** In the early stages, ovarian cancer is usually asymptomatic. Clinical manifestations may include general abdominal discomfort (gas, indigestion, pressure, bloating, cramps), sense of pelvic heaviness, loss of appetite, feeling of fullness, and change in bowel habits. As the malignancy grows, a variety of manifestations can occur, such as increase in abdominal girth, bowel and bladder dysfunction, persistent pelvic or abdominal pain, menstrual irregularities, and ascites. Palpation of a pelvic mass is usually the first assessment finding.

4. **Discuss diagnostic studies to confirm ovarian cancer.** An abdominal or vaginal ultrasound can be used to detect ovarian masses. A color Doppler imaging in conjunction with ultrasonography can be used to visualize vascular changes associated with malignancy and can determine if the mass is solid or cystic. If the woman is at high risk, a combination of tumor marker, CA-125, and ultrasound is recommended in addition to an annual pelvic examination. CA-125 is positive in 80% of women with epithelial ovarian cancer and is used to monitor the course of the disease. Lysophosphatidic acid (LPA), for which there is a new diagnostic blood test, functions to stimulate the growth of ovarian cancer. Therefore, elevated levels of LPA would be positive for ovarian cancer.

The following are prescribed:

- Transfuse with one unit of PRBC, repeat Hct after one hour. If Hct is below 30%, transfuse with the second unit of PRBC.
- Diphenhydramine HcL (Benadryl) 50 mg IM before starting paclitaxel
- Cisplatin (Platinol) 100 mg/m^2 once q three to four times a week
- Paclitaxel (Taxol) IV 135 mg/m^2 24-h infusion repeat q22days
- Aprepitant (Emend) 125 mg PO one hour prior to chemotherapy then 80 mg every AM for two days

5. **What are the purposes for the prescribed orders?** The PRBCs transfusion increases the hematocrit and hemoglobin levels by expanding blood volume. A repeat Hct is done to determine if the one unit of PRBC is sufficient to increase the Hct to at least 37%, which is in the range of normal Hct for a female adult. If the Hct level has not reached within the normal range, the second unit will be given. Another reason the Hct needs to be within the normal range is that Mrs. E is bleeding heavily and will need replenishing of blood volume. *Benadryl* prevents the allergic reaction that could occur from paclitaxel. *Benadryl* blocks histamine release by competing for H$_1$ receptor sites on effector cells. *Cisplatin* and *paclitaxel* eradicate cancer cells. *Paclitaxel* destroys cancer cells by interfering with the growth of rapidly dividing cells including cancer cells. Cancer cell death occurs because *paclitaxel* interferes with the microtubule network that is essential for cell interphase and cell mitosis. This interference eventually causes death of abnormal cells. Working in combination (synergy) with *cisplatin*, both drugs are effective throughout the entire cell cycle. *Cisplatin* is an antineoplastic, alkylating agent that produces interstrand and intrastrand cross linkage in DNA of rapidly dividing cells, thus preventing DNA and RNA

protein synthesis, which slows the progression of the disease process and eventually causes cell death. *Aprepitant* prevents acute and delayed nausea and vomiting by occupying brain NK_1 receptors and NK_1 receptors in the gastrointestinal (GI) system. *Aprepitant* is administered because *cisplatin* is a highly emetogenic drug, with nausea and vomiting beginning about one hour after administration and persisting for one to two days. *Aprepitant* is a selective receptor antagonist with two substances in its makeup: substance P and substance NK-1 receptors that are present in areas in the brain that control the emetic reflex. It is effective because it crosses the blood-brain barrier and occupies the brain NK_1 receptor.

6. What are the most common adverse reactions, drug-to-drug, drug-to-food/herbal interactions of the prescribed medications? The most common adverse reactions of *benadryl* are marked drowsiness, tachycardia, dry mouth, and anorexia. Drug-to-drug interactions may occur with the simultaneous use of other antihistamines, alcohol, opioid analgesics, and sedative/hypnotics, which increases the risk of central nervous system (CNS) depression. The simultaneous use of tricyclic antidepressants, quinidine, or disopyramide increases anticholinergic reactions. Monoamine oxidase (MAO) inhibitors intensify and prolong the anticholinergic effects of antihistamines. Drug-to-herbal interactions may occur with the simultaneous use of kava, valerian, or chamomile, which can increase CNS depression. The most common adverse reactions of *cisplatin* are ototoxicity, tinnitus, severe nausea, nausea, vomiting, hypocalcemia, hypokalemia, and hypomagnesemia. Drug-to-drug interactions may occur with the simultaneous use of aminoglycosides and amphotericin B, increasing the risk of nephrotoxicity, hypokalemia, hypomagnesemia, and acute renal failure. The simultaneous use of loop diuretics such as furosemide increase the risk of ototoxicity. The simultaneous use of phenytoin decreases phenytoin levels, and increased bone marrow depression may occur with other antineoplastic or radiation therapy. Cisplatin may decrease antibody response to live-virus vaccine and increase adverse reactions. There are no clinically significant drug-to-food/herbal interactions established. The most common adverse reactions of *paclitaxel* are transient bradycardia, peripheral neuropathy, nausea, vomiting, mucositis, anemia, hypersensitivity reactions, urticaria, abdominal and extremity pain, diaphoresis, myalgia, diarrhea, alopecia, leukopenia, thrombocytopenia, and arthralgias. Drug-to-drug interactions may occur with the simultaneous use of cisplatin and doxorubicin, which may increase myelosuppression. The simultaneous use of ketoconazoe, cyclosporine, doxorubicin, felodipine, diazepam, and midazolam may decrease paclitaxel metabolism. The simultaneous use of anticoagulants and nonsteroidal anti-inflammatory agents (NSAIDs) may enhance bleeding. Myelosuppression increases when given after *cisplatin.* The simultaneous use with doxorubicin may increase levels and toxicity of doxorubicin. There are no

clinically significant drug-to-food/herbal interactions established. The most common adverse reactions of *aprepitant* are fatigue, constipation, diarrhea, anorexia, nausea, and hiccups. Drug-to-drug interactions may occur with the simultaneous use of docetaxel, paclitaxel, etoposide, irinotecan, ifosfamide, imatinib, vinorelbine, vinblastine, vincristine, midazolam, triazolam, aprazolam, dofetilide, pimozide, phenobarbital, and warfarin may increase cause toxic effects. Drug-to-food interactions may occur with the simultaneous use of grapefruit juice, which may decrease the effectiveness of *aprepitant*. Drug-to-herbal interaction may occur with the simultaneous use of St. John's Wort, which may decrease the effectiveness of *aprepitant*.

7. **Describe the various staging done with ovarian cancer.** **Stage 0** indicates that the tumor is in situ, and treatment may include cervical conization, cryosurgery, or laser surgery. **Stage I** refers to strict confinement to the cervix, and treatment would be the same as for stage 0. **Stage IA** is microinvasive and the treatment involves radiation or surgery. **Stage IB** is similar to stage IA. **Stage II** refers to extension beyond the cervix but not to the pelvic wall, with involvement of the vagina but not as far as the lower third. **Stage IIA** has no obvious parametrial involvement, and **Stage IIB** has obvious parametrial involvement. The treatment is with radiation, hysterectomy, or pelvic exenteration. **Stage III** refers to extension to pelvic wall, no cancer-free space between tumor and pelvic wall on rectal examination. There is involvement of lower third of vagina, hydronephrosis, or nonfunctioning kidney. Radiation therapy is the treatment. **Stage IIIA** has no extension to pelvic wall, and **Stage IIIB** has extension to pelvic wall, hydronephrosis, or nonfunctioning kidney and may require radiation. **Stage IV** has extension beyond true pelvis or clinical involvement of the mucosa of bladder or rectum. The treatment is radiation or surgery. **Stage IVA** has spread to adjacent organs, and **Stage IVB** has spread to distant organs. Treatment is radiation or surgery, or combination of radiation and surgery.

8. **Discuss surgical management of ovarian malignancy.** A borderline malignancy may be treated conservatively with a total hysterectomy with bilateral salpingo-oopherectomy (TAH-BSO), the removal of urterus, cervix, fallopian tubes, and ovaries. This procedure can be done vaginally or abdominally. Primary complications that may occur post-surgery are hemorrhage and infection.

9. **Discuss client education for ovarian cancer.** Clients with family history of gynecological cancers and who have increased genetic risks should see their gynecological health care provider annually. Mrs. E has a strong family history of gynecologic and breast cancer and probably did not know enough about the genetic trait of the disease to seek counseling. Genetic counseling, like all other types of counseling, is confidential and helps

families to identify their cancer risks and to take steps that help reduce their risks before screening is done. *Menorrhagia* is the medical term for excessive or prolonged bleeding, or both. It is also referred to as hypermenorrhea. Some causes of menorrhagia is related to hormonal imbalance, such as a balance between estrogen and progesterone, which work together to create a balance. Excessive or prolonged bleeding can lead to other medical conditions such as hypovolemic shock and should be reported promptly.

10. Explain clinical implications for ovarian cancer. Paclitaxel is extremely water insoluble (hydrophobic), and for this reason, it is put into a solution containing oil rather than water. The particular oil is a type of castor oil called Cremophor EL, the same oil in which cyclosporin is mixed and that many clients cannot tolerate, and if taken shows hypersensitivity reactions similar to anaphylactic reactions. It is for this reason that, before clients receive paclitaxel, they are premedicated with a steroid, antihistamine, and an H_2 antagonist (cimetidine, ranitidine, famotidine, or nizatidine). The drug must be administered under the supervision of an experienced oncology nurse, NP, or health care provider.

References

Black, J. M. and Hawks, J. H. (2005). *Medical-Surgical Nursing: Clinical Management for Positive Outcomes*. Philadelphia: W. B. Saunders.

Broyles, B. E. (2005). *Medical-Surgical Nursing Clinical Companion*. Durham, NC: Carolina Academic Press.

Corbet, J. V. (2004). *Laboratory Tests and Diagnostic Procedures with Nursing Diagnoses* (6th ed.). Upper Saddle River, NJ: Prentice Hall.

Flemm, L. A. (June 2004). "Aprepitant for Chemotherapy-Induced Nausea and Vomiting." *Clinical Journal of Oncology Nursing* 8(3): 303–306.

Gahart, B. L. and Nazareno, A. R. (2005). *2005 Intravenous Medications*. St. Louis: Mosby.

Zanotti, K. (May 2002). "Gynecologic Malignancies: Endometrial, Ovarian, and Cervical Cancer." Available at www.clevelandclinicmeded.com/diseasemanagement/women/gynmalignancy/gynmalignancy.htm.

Huether, S. E. and McCance, K. L. (2004). *Understanding Pathophysiology* (3rd ed.). St. Louis: Mosby.

Ignatavicius, D. D. and Workman, M. L. (2006). *Medical-Surgical Nursing across the Health Care Continuum* (5th ed.). Philadelphia: W. B. Saunders.

Spratto, G. R. and Woods, A. L. (2005). *2005 Edition: PDR Nurse's Drug Handbook*. Clifton Park, NY: Thomson Delmar Learning.

CASE STUDY 3

Rheumatoid Arthritis

GENDER

F

AGE

52

SETTING

- Home

ETHNICITY/CULTURE

- Black American/West Indian descent

PREEXISTING CONDITIONS

COEXISTING CONDITIONS

- Father has RA

LIFESTYLE

- Ordained minister
- Early retirement as laboratory technician

COMMUNICATION

DISABILITY

- Pain in the hands and lower extremities

SOCIOECONOMIC STATUS

- Low

SPIRITUAL/RELIGIOUS

- Methodist

PHARMACOLOGIC

- Hydroxychloroquine sulfate (Plaquenil)
- Methotrexate (Rheumatrex Dose Pack)
- Ibuprofen (Motrin)
- Ranitidine HcL (Zantac)
- Minocycline (Minocin)

PSYCHOSOCIAL

- Anxiety
- Periods of depression

LEGAL

- Persons with RA should qualify for disability benefits through the federal Social Security program.

ETHICAL

ALTERNATIVE THERAPY

- Cold-water fish
- Fish oil capsules
- Vitamins C and E

PRIORITIZATION

- Pain management

DELEGATION

- RN
- Client education

MODERATE

THE MUSCULOSKELETAL AND REPRODUCTIVE SYSTEMS

Level of difficulty: High

Overview: This case involves a thorough assessment of the client's psychosocial status to detect subtle signs of depression and intervene appropriately and immediately. It also involves thorough assessment of the client's condition, including identifying typical patterns of joint involvement, palpating tissues around joints to elicit pain or tenderness, and eliciting of prescribed and nonprescribed drugs and herbal therapy. It also involves a nurse who is more supportive than assertive, which will help the client view her illness in a more positive manner with hope for improvement.

Client Profile

Ms. D is a 52-year-old single female who is admitted to the hospital due to moderate weight loss, fever, and extreme fatigue over the past two weeks. She is 5'9" and weighs 140 pounds. Her vital signs are:

Blood pressure: 150/92
Pulse: 88
Respirations: 20
Temperature: 101.6° F

Case Study

On initial interview, Ms. D reports family history of rheumatoid arthritis, which she believes is directly related to the paternal side of the family. Continued discussion reveals that Ms. D had two previous episodes of suicidal ideation, which are documented in records brought with her to the hospital. Her document indicates that the suicidal ideations were related to periods of depression due to early retirement and unemployment secondary to inability to use upper extremities to perform required tasks at her place of employment. Past medical history reveals pneumonia and pericarditis. Ms. D's chief complaints on admission are severe morning stiffness, especially of the digits of both hands, that lasts for more than one hour upon waking. History and physical by the chief resident finds joints of the upper extremities to be soft and very painful to touch, with fluid evident in the joints of upper extremities and bilateral knees. Serum labs reveal:

Albumin: 6 g/dl
Alpha globulin: 1 g/dl
White blood cell (WBC) count: $16,000/mm^3$
Hematocrit (Hct): 26.8%
Platelets count (PLT): $525,000/mm^3$
Calcium: 7.8 mg/dL
Granulocyte: 82.8%
Lymphocyte: 8.8%

Also revealed are the presence of antinuclear antibodies, decreased C4 complement component, elevated C-reactive protein, and elevated erythrocyte sedimentation rate (ESR). The Rose-Waaler test is positive, the client is seropositive, and immunoglobulin G (IgG) is elevated. Bone X-ray of the upper and lower extremities reveals minimal joint involvement, and a magnetic resonance imaging (MRI) of the spine reveals beginning spinal column disease. An arthrocentesis is done, and the synovial fluid is positive for inflammatory cells, immune complexes, and rheumatoid factor (RF). A diagnosis of rheumatoid arthritis is confirmed. Ms. D is placed on bed rest and an order for physical therapy is written.

Questions

1. Discuss pathophysiology, incidence, prevalence, and risk factors of RA.

2. Discuss clinical manifestations of RA.

3. Discuss the extra-articular manifestations of RA.

4. Discuss the management of advanced, unremitting RA.

5. What are the purposes for the prescribed orders?

6. What are the most common adverse reactions, drug-to-drug, drug-to-food/herbal interactions for the prescribed medications?

7. Discuss nonpharmacologic modalities for RA management.

8. Discuss client education for RA.

Questions and Suggested Answers

1. Discuss pathophysiology, incidence, prevalence, and risk factors of RA.
RA is a chronic, systemic autoimmune disorder whose major distinctive feature is chronic, symmetrical, and erosive inflammation of the synovial tissue of the joints. The severity of the joint disease may fluctuate over time, but progressive development of various degrees of joint destruction, deformity, and disability are the most common outcomes of established disease. The presence of RF, an autoantibody directed against IgG is found in more than 80% of clients with the disease. There is also the identification of antibodies against collagen, Epstein-Barr virus, encoded nuclear antigen, and certain other antigens. RA occurs worldwide and affects all racial and ethnic groups. It can occur at any time of life, but its incidence tends to increase with age, peaking between the fourth and sixth decades. Women are affected more than men. The prevalence rates for black Americans is similar to that of white Americans. Gene mutations are associated with RA, especially if they are present in a person with varieties of the tissue type human leukocyte antigen (HLA)-DRB, HLA-DR4, or HLA-DP. A genetic predisposition for RA is seen in identical twins, but the strongest genetic evidence is seen in the association of RA with HLA-DR4, a genetically determined allele. The primary joint lesions involve the *synovium*. With the initial formation of immune complexes, synovitis develops as the synovial membrane becomes swollen, irritated, and inflamed. Immune complexes are deposited onto the synovial membrane or the superficial layers of the articular cartilage; they are phagocytized by polymorphonuclear (PMN) leukocytes, monocytes, and lymphocytes. Phagocytosis deactivates the immune complexes and simultaneously produces additional enzymes that lead to hyperemia, edema, swelling, and thickening of the synovial lining. The hypertrophied synovium invades the surrounding tissue, including cartilage, ligaments, joint capsule, and tendons. Eventually, granulation tissue forms to cover the entire articular cartilage, leading to the formation

of *pannus*, a highly vascularized fibrous scar tissue composed of lymphocytes, macrophages, histiocytes, fibroblasts, and mast cells. Pannus is the most destructive element in RA and can erode and destroy articular cartilage, which will eventually result in subchondral bone erosions, bone cysts, fissures, and development of bone spurs and osteophytes. Pannus can also scar and shorten tendons and ligaments, conditions that lead to ligamentous laxity, subluxation, and contractures.

2. **Discuss clinical manifestations of RA.** The clinical manifestations of RA vary, usually reflecting the stage and severity of the disease. Joint pain, swelling, warmth, erythema, and lack of function are classic manifestations. Characteristically, the pattern of joint involvement begins with the small joints in the hands, wrists, and feet. In the early stages of the disease, limitation in function can occur when there is active inflammation in the joints. The client tends to guard or protect these joints through immobilization. Deformity of feet and hands are common due to misalignment resulting from swelling, progressive joint destruction, or the subluxation (partial dislocation) that occurs when a bone slips over another and eliminates the joint space. Carpal tunnel syndrome, the compression of the median nerve as a result of tenosynovitis on the volar aspect of the wrists, is fairly common. "Cock-up toes" result from plantar subluxation of the metatarsal heads. Popliteal cysts (*Baker's cysts*) can develop behind the knee joint.

3. **Discuss the extra-articular manifestations of RA.** The three most frequent extra-articular manifestations of RA are Sjogren's syndrome, Felty's syndrome, and Caplan's syndrome. *Sjogren's syndrome* is an immunologic disorder characterized by deficient fluid production by the lacrimal, salivary,

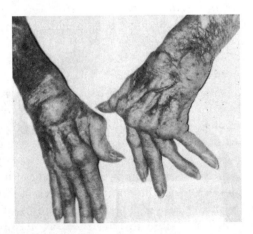

Rheumatoid arthritis

and other mucous membranes. Atrophy of the lacrimal glands can lead to desiccation of the cornea and conjunctiva with damage to the tissues. Atrophy of the salivary glands results in dental disorders and loss of taste and odor sensations. When the lungs are affected, the dryness increases susceptibility to pneumonia and other respiratory infections. Treatment involves artificial tears, using soft contact lenses, sipping fluids frequently to prevent mouth dryness, and avoiding medications that tend to deplete body fluids. *Felty's syndrome* is a group of pathologic changes that occur with adult RA characterized by splenomegaly, leukopenia, frequent infections, and sometimes thrombocytopenia and anemia. Surgical resection of the spleen often temporarily improves the condition of the enlarged spleen. *Caplan's syndrome* is evidenced with pneumoconiosis, with symptoms of RA, and radiographic evidence of intrapulmonary nodules.

4. Discuss the management of advanced, unremitting RA. For advanced, unremitting RA, immunosuppressive agents are prescribed because of their ability to affect the production of antibodies at the cellular level. The medication regimen includes high-dose methotrexate, cyclophosphamide, and azathioprine. However, because these medications are highly toxic and can produce bone marrow suppression, anemia, gastrointestinal (GI) disturbances, and rashes, nurses must be vigilant with monitoring when these medications are administered. The FDA has approved a device, a protein "A" immunoadsorption column (Prosorba), which is used in 12 weekly apheresis treatments to bind IgG (circulating immune complex).

The following are prescribed:

- Hydroxychloroquine sulfate (Plaquenil) 200 mg PO two times per day
- Methotrexate (Rheumatrex Dose Pack) 2.5 mg q12h for three doses each week
- Ibuprofen (Motrin) 400 mg PO three times per day
- Ranitidine HcL (Zantac) 150 mg every night at bedtime
- Minocycline HcL (Minocin) 100 mg PO q12h

5. What are the purposes for the prescribed orders? *Hydroxychloroquine sulfate* is an antirheumatic (DMARDs) and antimalarial agent that decreases the inflammatory process in RA, but the mechanism by which it decreases the inflammatory process is unknown. *Methotrexate* is classified as an antimetabolite antineoplastic that, when used for RA, acts by inhibiting dihydrofolate reductase, resulting in the decreased synthesis of purines, and functions to decrease the immune process believed to be involved in the autoimmune process of RA. *Ibuprofen* is a nonsteroidal anti-inflammatory (NSAID) agent that decreases the inflammatory process associated with RA activity. *Ranitidine* is a histamine H-2 receptor blocking agent used for heartburn and gastric irritation associated with the use of ibuprofen. *Minocycline*

HcL is a broad-spectrum antibiotic used to slow the anti-inflammatory process with mechanisms recently discovered but not yet understood.

6. **What are the most common adverse reactions, drug-to-drug, drug-to-food/herbal interactions for the prescribed medications?** The most common adverse reaction of *hydroxychloroquine sulfate* is retinopathy. Drug-to-drug interactions may occur with the simultaneous use of *hydroxychloroquine* and hepatotoxic drugs such as acetaminophen, which may increase the risk of liver toxicity. When used concurrently with digoxin, hydroxychloroquine increases serum digoxin levels. The simultaneous use with penicillamine may increase the risk of hematologic toxicity. Use with either magnesium-based or aluminum-based antacids decreases the action of hydroxychloroquine. There are no drug-to-food/herbal interactions established. The most common adverse effects of *methotrexate* include bone marrow depression, hepatotoxicity, acne, cheymosis, and increased pigmentation. With *methotrexate* drug-to-drug interactions may occur with the simultaneous use of alcohol, azathioprine, etretinate, doxycycline, and sulfasalazine, increasing the risk of hepatotoxicity. Oral aminoglycocides, antacids, and chloramphenicol decrease the absorption of oral methotrexate. Ingesting more than 180 mg of caffeine per day may decrease the effects of methotrexate. When used in conjunction with anticoagulants, there is an increased risk of hypoprothrombinemia. Ibuprofen, PABA, probenecid, pyrimethamine, salicylates, tetracyclines, and vancomycin increase the effects of methotrexate. Also sulfonamides and trimethoprim increase the risks of bone marrow suppression. Further, methotrexate decreases serum digoxin levels if used concurrently with digoxin. No clinically significant drug-to-food/herbal interactions have been established. The most common adverse reactions of *ibuprofen* are headache, constipation, dyspepsia, nausea, and vomiting. Drug-to-drug interactions may occur with the simultaneous use of low-dose aspirin, which may limit the cardioprotective effects of aspirin. Additive adverse GI side effects may occur with the simultaneous use of *ibuprofen* with aspirin, NSAIDs, corticosteroids, or alcohol. Simultaneous use of *ibuprofen* and diuretics or antihypertensives may decrease their effects. The simultaneous use with insulin or oral hypoglycemic agents may increase hypoglycemic effects. The concurrent use with digoxin, lithium, methotrexate, probenecid with *ibuprofen* will increase risk of toxicity. Increased risk of bleeding will be seen if *ibuprofen* is used simultaneously with cefamandole, cefotetan, cefoperazone, valproic acid, plicamycin, thrombolytic agents, warfarin, and drugs affecting platelet function such as clopidogrel bisulfate, ticlopidine, abciximab, eptifibatide, or tirofiban. The simultaneous use of *ibupofren* and antineoplastics or radiation therapy increases the risk of adverse hematologic reactions, and its use with cyclosporine increases the risk of nephrotoxicity. Drug-to-food interactions

are not clinically established, however most clients should take ibuprofen with food to decrease the gastric irritation. Drug-to-herbal interactions occurs with the simultaneous use of anise, arnica, chamomile, clove, dong, quai, feenugreek, feverfew, garlic, ginger, gingko, Panax ginseng, and licorice. The most common adverse effects associated with *ranitidine HcL* include constipation, diarrhea, headache, and dizziness, and it can cause psychogenic effects. The most common adverse reactions of *minocycline HcL* are dizziness, vestibular reactions, diarrhea, nausea, vomiting, and photo-sensitivity. Drug-to-drug interactions can occur with the simultaneous use of *ranitidine HcL* and antacids that may decrease ranitidine absorption. Currently no clinically significant drug-to-food/herbal interactions have been established. Drug-to-drug interactions may occur with the simultaneous use of *minocycline HcL* and barbiturates, carbamazepine, phenytoin, penicillins, and oral contraceptives may decrease the effects of these agents, whereas use with warfarin may increase the effect of warfarin. The simultaneous use of *minocycline HcL* with antacids, calcium, zinc, kaolin and pectin, sodium bicarbonate, iron, and magnesium decrease the absorption of minocycline HcL. The simultaneous use with bismuth subsalicylate can significantly decrease *minocycline HcL* absorption. If *minocycline HcL* is taken with dairy products, its absorption will be greatly increased. There are no clinically established drug-to-herbal interactions.

7. Discuss nonpharmacologic modalities for RA management. Non-pharmacologic management for RA includes adequate rest, which includes local, systemic, and psychological rest. In *local rest* a joint is immobilized with a splint or brace, and if the joint is inflamed, it is rested until the inflammation subsides. *Systemic rest* involves immobilization of the entire body, such as during a nap. The client should try to sleep for eight to ten hours and, if possible, rest an additional one to two hours each day. *Psychological rest* involves removing oneself from the daily stresses that can enhance pain. The client can use relaxation therapies such as meditation, imagery, or music to induce relaxation and reduce stress.

8. Discuss client education for RA. The client should balance activity with rest by taking naps during the day. The client should pace him- or herself to avoid planning too much for one day. The client should set priorities by determining which activities are most important, and do those first. The client should delegate responsibility and tasks to others in the home. The client should plan ahead to prevent last-minute rushing and stress, and should know his or her own activity tolerance and not exceed it. Both ver-bal and written information concerning the medications, dosages, adverse effects, and frequency of taking the agents should be provided. Range-of-motion exercises and use of assistive or adaptive devices should be explained as well as providing information concerning support groups for those with RA. The nurse should stress the importance of follow-up care with the client and explain all referrals prescribed.

References

Corbett. J. V. (2004). *Laboratory Tests and Diagnostic Procedures with Nursing Diagnoses* (6th ed). Upper Saddle River, NJ: Prentice Hall.

Deglin, J. H. and Vallerand, A. H. (2005). *Davis's Drug Guide for Nurses* (9th ed.). Philadelphia: F. A. Davis.

Drugs @ FDA. Available at www.assessdata.fda.gov.

Ignatavicius, D. D. and Workman, M. L. (2006). *Medical-Surgical Nursing across the Health Care Continuum* (5th ed.). Philadelphia: W. B. Saunders.

"Rheumatoid Arthritis and the Diet Alternative." (January 2006). Available at www.paleodiet.com/ra.

Rupp, I., Boshuizen, H. C., Jacobi, C. E., Dinant, H. J., and van den Bos, G. A. M. (January 2004). "Comorbidity in Patients with Rheumatoid Arthritis: Effect on Health-Related Quality of Life." *Journal of Rheumatology* 31(1): 58–62.

Skidmore-Roth, L. (2006). *Mobsy's Handbook of Herbs & Natural Supplements* (3rd ed.). St. Louis: Mosby.

Spratto, G. R. and Woods, A. L. (2005). *2005 Edition: PDR Nurse's Drug Handbook*. Clifton Park, NY: Thomson Delmar Learning.

Index